Cracking the Beauty Code

HOW TO PROGRAM YOUR DNA FOR HEALTH, VITALITY, AND YOUNGER-LOOKING SKIN

Cracking the Beauty Code

HOW TO PROGRAM YOUR DNA FOR HEALTH, VITALITY, AND YOUNGER-LOOKING SKIN

Dr. Anne Marie Fine

Fine Natural Products, LLC
NEWPORT BEACH, CA

Fine Natural Product, LLC
280 Cagney Ln #317
Newport Beach, CA 92663

www.drannemariefine.com

Ordering Information:

Quantity sales. Special discounts are available on quantity purchases by corporations, associations, and others. For details, contact the "Special Sales Department" at the address above.

Cracking the Beauty Code, Dr. Anne Marie Fine —1st ed.

ISBN 978-0-9986493-0-6

Book Layout ©2017 www.BrightFlameBooks.com

Contents

Disclaimer

This book contains the opinions and ideas of its author. It is intended to provide helpful general information on the subjects it addresses. It is not in any way a substitute for the advice of a reader's own physician(s) or other medical professionals based on the reader's own individual conditions, symptoms, or concerns. If the reader needs personal medical, health, dietary, exercise, or other assistance or advice, the reader should consult a competent physician and/or other qualified health care professionals. The author specifically disclaims all responsibility for injury, damage, or loss that the reader may incur as a direct or indirect consequence of following any directions or suggestions given in the book or participating in any programs described in the book.

Introduction

HAVE YOU EVER WONDERED why some people look better for their age than others? Many people believe this is simply due to genetics, or less exposure to the sun, the most well-known skin ager. And yet, there is more to it than simply genetics or sun exposure. Recent scientific advances demonstrate that our environment exerts significantly more control over genes than was previously thought. In fact, it is being shown that our environment is the software that is driving our DNA hardware—a revolutionary concept called epigenetics. We now know that our epigenome (the sum total of our environment) is able to turn on or off our genes and play important roles in stem cell differentiation, hair growth and rates of graying, wound healing, inflammation, hyper- and hypopigmentation, DNA repair, aging, cell longevity, and skin diseases such as eczema, psoriasis, and vitiligo. What's even more astonishing is that epigenetic mechanisms regulate our own body's production of endogenous antioxidants.

Epigenetics speaks to the very underpinnings of the "Beauty from Within" trend, and holds the potential to define the influences of our environment not only on our skin, but on our entire aging process as well. This is the future of not only skin care but also of medicine!

This book is packed with dozens of unique strategies to radically transform your skin into an age-defying masterpiece that glows with true radiance and beauty simply by changing our environment; in particular, diet and lifestyle. At the same time, these strategies work at the genomic level to retard aging on the inside, too. It is entirely possible to be one chronological age and a completely different biological age.

Most of us accept skin aging as a normal process of aging and that, beyond the techniques offered by dermatologists and plastic surgeons, nothing else can be done about it. This book will break through and dispel these myths of aging and reveal the causes of visible signs of aging that can be mitigated. This is done through a concept called "beauty from the inside out," where nutrition, stress, lifestyle, environmental toxicants, emotional milieu, and digestion are all contributing "environmental" factors in the aging of the skin.

Beauty is an inside job. You really are what you eat and what you think, breathe, and drink, too. And nowhere is this more evident than on your skin, which is merely a reflection of your overall health. In fact, it is impossible to have truly radiant skin without also being truly healthy. Many of my patients who have come to see me over the years with diverse skin conditions, such as psoriasis, eczema, atopic dermatitis, acne, rashes, bumps, rosacea, age spots, dryness, dull skin, premature aging, and more, have been treated to dramatic skin transformation through health restoration. In fact, when a new patient comes to see me, I can learn a lot about that person's health by simply observing the skin. The condition of your skin is a clue to what is going on inside your body.

We're in the midst of probably the biggest revolution in biology that is going to forever transform the way we understand genetics, environment, the way the two interact, what causes disease, what contributes to health, and even what causes different rates of aging. It's another level of biology, which, for the first time really, is up to the task of explaining the sheer physiological complexity of life. Let me explain this further by going back in time.

When the Human Genome Project was completed in 2003, it was hoped that this ambitious project would yield cures for most diseases and practical applications in biotechnology to improve lives. While there have been some important products from this endeavor, and assuredly more to come, what is more interesting is that many genes thought to be responsible for some diseases, in fact, only account for a mere fraction of that disease. For example, in the case of breast cancer, much excitement was generated with the discovery of the BRCA 1 and BRCA 2 genes—the so-called breast cancer genes. However, less than 10% of women with breast cancer have these genes, meaning more than 90% of breast cancer is caused by environmental factors. These environmental factors are epigenetic factors—they act on the DNA turning certain genes on and off.

Natural molecules found in food and supplements influence hundreds and even thousands of genes. Vitamin D is a good example of this as it is widely believed to influence 2,000 different genes. This means that the food you eat speaks directly to your genes. In fact, your entire environment is having a conversation with your entire genome 24 hours a day. Your DNA is literally bathed constantly in a sea of information deriving from the food you eat, the supplements you take, your thoughts, emotional milieu, and your exposure to environmental toxins. These factors are powerful regulators of your health as they turn on and off the genes that are either promoting health and vitality or aging us and sending us down the pathway of poor health.

Incredibly, only about two percent of diseases can be attributed to locked-in, single-gene mutations. Most disease occurs as a complex interaction between genetic susceptibility and the environment. This means, while there are genetic predispositions, there are environmental triggers that actually start the disease, and also environmental factors that protect against developing the disease. The key is to understand which factors promote disease and avoid them, and which factors protect and seek them out. Our genetic makeup doesn't necessarily determine our biological fate, although it can certainly predispose.

As a doctor focusing on environmental medicine, I have taken a careful look at the environmental factors that influence skin. And I have found that our environment is really impactful with respect to our skin health and how we age. This book is my way of sharing this positive message: that we have considerably more control over the aging process than we once thought.

The intent of this book is to get us beyond "what new beauty product can I try that will improve how I look" and the whole "anti-aging" perspective that attempts to resist the natural passage of time. It's time to embrace aging (because the alternative is being dead), but also understand that slowing the visible signs of aging is possible and will result in retarding aging on the inside, too. We want to LOOK and FEEL healthy and vibrant!

Wisdom, strength, and health are the new buzzwords for aging and beauty. Healthy is the new beautiful!

The book is based on the premise of 6 Critical Concepts for turning on your beauty genes:

- Eating for Beauty
- Supplements for Beauty
- Detoxification for Beauty
- Emotional Well-being for Beauty
- Sleeping for Beauty
- Clean Products for Beauty

At the end of each chapter, I will present three different levels of interventions for you to incorporate into your life. I recognize that all of you will have different motivation, time, energy, and money with which to make changes in your lives, and all of you are at different places in your lives as well.

The first level is the **Minimalist.** This is the person who wants the biggest change for her buck, or time, and doesn't have a lot of resources or patience to do it all, because she is already doing it all somewhere else. If this is you, I celebrate you for having personal awareness of what would work for you.

The second level is the **Middle Way.** This is the person who wishes to see a bigger change and is willing to put in the time, energy, and money to do so.

The third level is the **Beauty Buff.** This person is seeking to overcome previous damage to her skin and/or puts a high priority on beauty and has the motivation, money, and time to go full-out to reap the rewards of these changes.

At the end of the book, I have created the 21-Day IAMFINE® Protocol for Facial Rejuvenation, in case you prefer to follow an established plan instead of incorporating a few ideas at a time.

CHAPTER ONE

How Skin Ages

"We are what we eat, drink, breathe, believe, and think, and we simply cannot medicate a patient out of faulty diet or lifestyle."
—Dr. Fine

BEAUTY AND WELLNESS ARE INTERTWINED and, at this point in time, they are converging in a complex landscape where nutrition, beauty, fitness, spirituality, and emotional wellbeing coalesce holistically to make us whole. As our population ages, many strategies are being discovered and marketed to promote overall health and wellbeing that will reflect externally as more youthful-looking skin. Healthy-eating patterns and other lifestyle choices have been linked to resilience against age-related decline. People are living longer, working longer, and wish to continue enjoying all of their activities well into old age. They fervently desire to maintain their attractive looks and youthful energy levels as they age.

At the same time we are enjoying a full-blown revolution in the area of genetics. Medical scientists have revealed that only a minority of our diseases are fully caused by genes, leaving the rest due to the complex interplay between our environment and our genes; this is called epigenetics. Even more surprising is the news that hereditary factors, i.e., our genes, only affect about 25% of our age at death or our longevity.

Our skin is especially vulnerable and responsive to aging damage both from the outside-in and the inside-out. Rapid skin-cell turnover and production requires a constant supply of the appropriate nutrients. Environmental factors, such as free radicals, pollution and toxins, humidity, and temperature can affect skin-barrier function while stress, poor nutrition, poor sleep, and inflammation can impair the skin's growth, maintenance, and ability to counteract outside forces.

That leaves a lot of room for choosing diet and lifestyle factors that favor a more healthy aging. We are beginning to discover that we have some control and mastery over our life's masterpiece: us. We now can embrace this new model and truly transform our health in order to become the best version of ourselves that we can be. The phrase "Genes may load the gun, but environment pulls the trigger," is commonly heard in the environmental medicine arena.

This book examines skin in a new way, laying out the real reasons why your skin ages and illuminating what can be done about it through conscious choices in your diet and lifestyle. For example, sun damage is a well-known factor in skin aging. Applying sunscreen or staying out of the sun can be very helpful in preventing premature aging of the skin. The skin is amenable to easy, non-invasive changes that really can help you turn back the hands of time and grow older gracefully. At the same time, these choices will improve your health and wellbeing so that you can *feel* good, too. This book will also educate you on how to shop for clean personal care products so that you are not adding to your body's toxic burden and contributing to potential health problems.

My Story

Like many of you, I grew up in the sun unencumbered by hats, sunscreen, and special clothes with SPF embedded in the fabric. I had not a care in the world as I played tennis nearly every day, ran outside, and frolicked at the beach. Growing up in Newport Beach, California, we teenage girls thought the sun was providing us with a great makeup trick: if our faces were tan enough, we could forego the foundation in our makeup routines.

We strove to keep up our tans, even applying baby oil and other regrettable substances on our skin to enhance our "glow." Even the sunscreen that was available at the time said on its label Suntan Lotion—an obvious nod to the fact that while a blazing red sunburn that blistered was not cool, enough sun to create a tan certainly was.

We did notice that the lifeguards on their lifeguard stands stood out with their zinc oxide-encrusted noses. I always wondered what that stuff was, and thought that the white nose totally detracted from their overall bronzed, muscular beauty. As a fair-skinned girl of Irish descent, I was always trying to dodge the inevitable sunburn and explosion of freckles while carefully layering on a nice tan. No one ever told me that sun exposure was the number one cause of premature skin aging! If only I had known. I was told that sun exposure could cause skin cancer later in life, but who really cares about that when you are a teenager and trying to be "cool"?

Fast-forward a few decades to when I had a life-changing experience with a Wood's lamp during medical school. A Wood's lamp is a piece of equipment that uses ultraviolet light to illuminate what is really going on underneath your skin. All the sun damage that is lurking underneath the visible portion of your skin, biding its time until it is revealed with age, is there for you and your doctor to see. This was a nauseating experience for me, especially since I had already added daily sunscreen to my skin-care program. There was so much damage lying in wait that I could easily envision the wrinkly, spotted visage that was surely in my future. To this day, I try to avoid looking at my face in a Wood's lamp.

This was a wake-up call, however; to see what I could do to take better care of my skin and possibly forestall some of these upcoming ravages of time. My interest in skin and natural skin care was ignited.

And what I discovered was truly amazing. Real, lasting skin health and rejuvenation largely comes from within, and inner health and radiance shines through to the outside. This book is not about makeup tricks or expensive trips to the dermatologist for "procedures," however well they work. I will share my wrinkle-transforming and wellness secrets with you in this book and point the way to true facial rejuvenation.

Gone are the days when I would not leave the house without makeup. I now wear makeup so seldom that my mascaras dry out long before I can get my money's worth out of them. My mother was right, why cover up gorgeous skin with a layer of makeup? But even more importantly, I feel healthier than when I was in my twenties and have overcome my other health challenges, which were far more damaging than sun-ravaged skin.

Now, my skin looks remarkably younger than my age in spite of my earlier cavalier attitude towards the sun. My son is often mistaken for my husband; my daughter for my sister. I decided to share what I learned about skin health, beauty, and wellness with my patients and a wider audience in order to help others prevent, reverse, and maintain their skin's natural beauty and age gracefully, gratefully, and healthfully.

Oh, I know there is a lot of help out there, everything from Botox, fillers, and lasers, to plastic surgery. But even these aesthetic techniques working their magic on the outside-in can benefit from skin that is healthier and more radiant from the inside-out. It is a win-win! And for the group of people who simply don't wish to undergo the "standard" route due to potential side effects, downtime, lack of interest, or money, my method stands alone. I wrote this book to empower all women (and men) to embrace their inner beauty naturally. I want to bring out the beauty in everyone!

At the same time, my interest in environmental medicine was piqued. I began to question why so many of my female patients had cancer, autoimmune disease, fibromyalgia, multiple chemical sensitivity, hormonal imbalances, and chronic fatigue syndrome. It seemed downright odd to me that nearly every woman in my practice suffered from some form of thyroid disease, including the autoimmune disease Hashimoto's Thyroiditis—a veritable epidemic in my practice. I began to wonder what was different between the women and men in my practice, and why the women were so much sicker. Then I realized that the sheer number of personal-care products women use every day could be a factor. I began to research and investigate the ingredients in some of the personal-care products that women use every day, sometimes multiple times per day. What I discovered was that some ingredients in skin-care products were not only NOT healthy for people, but were actually contributing to poor health.

I discovered that many of the commonly used ingredients in our personal-care products are endocrine disruptors, a class of substances that cause our hormones, including our thyroid hormones, to go out of balance. Other ingredients were exposed as carcinogens, neurotoxins, and reproductive toxins. In this book, I will explore this topic more fully, lay out the ingredients you want to avoid, and give you great tools to choose clean personal-care and beauty products for yourself and your families.

Of course, our exposure to environmental toxicants is not limited to personal-care products. We are also exposed through the food we eat, water we drink, air we breathe, and the very thoughts we think, but those are topics I explore in my other articles, blogs, and lectures.

This book examines skin in a new way, revealing the real reasons why your skin ages and illuminating what can be done about it through conscious choices in your diet and lifestyle. I have discovered that skin is amenable to easy, non-invasive changes that truly can help you turn back the hands of time and grow older gracefully. This book will also educate you on how to shop for clean personal-care products, so that you are not adding to your body's toxic burden and contributing to potential health problems.

Skin

Your skin is an amazing, yet underappreciated, organ of the body. It is actually the largest organ in the body and, completely spread out, takes up about 20 square feet. It does far more than just act as a protective barrier, although holding our insides in is a big job in itself. Your skin serves many functions, including that of an organ of elimination, temperature regulator, infection protector, vitamin-D synthesizer, and provider of sensory information to the brain regarding pain, tactile sensation, and pressure. Your skin is also the most visible indicator of the total health of your body, which is why, if you embrace certain positive health behaviors for the insides of your body, your skin will reward you by becoming clearer and more vibrant. Wrinkles will diminish, moisture content will improve, and texture will become more even.

The skin consists of two main parts: an outer layer called the epidermis and the layer below called the dermis.

The epidermis consists of four layers, from the top down: the stratum corneum, the stratum granulosum, stratum spinosum, and stratum basale. This fourth layer is the lowest level and the level at which the melanocytes live, the cells that make melanin, the pigment that colors your skin and functions as a protector of DNA from sun damage.

The epidermis is keratinized, stratified, squamous epithelium (essentially flattened dead skin cells) that provides chemical, physical, and mechanical protection as well as being the front line for any microbial infections. The primary cell type involved here is the keratinocyte, which makes keratin and other proteins, as well as lipid (fat) for the skin-barrier function of the epidermis. The other main cell type here is the dendritic cell, which is involved in immune function.

The skin-barrier function of our skin cannot be underestimated. The bricks and mortar scheme that alternates the keratin protein and lamellar fats has the job of keeping out certain environmental factors such as water. The skin-barrier function provides integrity and hydration of the skin by not allowing our internal water to evaporate from the skin very quickly. At the same time, it allows for other substances to penetrate. This is the basis of transdermal medications and hormones. It is also the reason why you want to be aware of what is being absorbed through your personal-care products, as research has shown certain ingredients from personal-use products can be absorbed systemically throughout our bodies.

Skin-barrier function is also involved in some skin diseases such as atopic dermatitis, eczema, and psoriasis. If skin barrier function is disrupted, many outside influences can make their way into the body more easily and that is why you see so many warning signs on products that say "do not apply to broken skin."

In the bottom layer, on the epidermis, the stratum basale, the skin's stem cells reside. These cells regulate epidermal renewal through keratinocyte development. Stem cells are the little beauty factories that you want to keep healthy and happy and producing radiant, newborn skin cells that will pop to the surface. These cells have also been found to be very responsive to epigenetic influences that lead to gene expression or repression. The stem cells respond to positive and negative outside factors and influence the quality of our skin.

New cells generated by the lower level of the epidermis are continuously being brought to the surface of the skin in order to replace the old cells that are being continuously shed. The very top layer of the epidermis, the stratum corneum, consists of these older skin cells. This process of skin turnover drastically decreases as we age and accounts for the loss of radiance in our skin as we get older. When we are young, this process usually only takes 30 days, but rises to 75 or more as we age. This is why proper exfoliation and peels can help restore radiance—they remove this top layer of cells. We lose the radiance because the top layer of our skin, the epidermis, becomes filled with old, crusty, dead skin cells that have not sloughed off yet.

The dermis itself is directly below the epidermis and provides scaffolding for strength and support. It is composed of an extracellular complex (ECM) containing collagen fibers whose primary function is to maintain firmness, elastin that provides skin elasticity, and various glycoproteins. The main cell type here is the fibroblast which is responsible for making the collagen, elastin, and other structural proteins that make up this layer. The dermis provides the cushioning in your skin and is also the place where the deep wrinkles reside. The formation of wrinkles results from impaired barrier function, loss of cells (skin thinning), and reduction of underlying structural proteins in the ECM, along with sugar-induced glycation of the same proteins.

Genes regulate these skin functions just as they regulate other bodily processes. In this book, I will discuss how certain strategies can result in a facial makeover by optimizing gene expression and DNA repair. This is the skin care of the twenty-first century, which allows us to leverage our knowledge of environmental and dietary influences on turning genes on and off for the purpose of thwarting Father

Time, and of aging in the most graceful way possible. Skin care and skin-care products are about to make a major change in order to utilize this huge paradigm shift in human health and aging. I expect we will see, in the near future, new skin-care products being developed that can target certain genes regulating skin function and aging for even better results on your skin.

The function of a gene is to make a protein, but something has to tell the genes when to turn on and produce a protein. A great analogy is that, in our bodies, genes are the hardware, but our environment is the software. The environment helps decide to turn on the genes that regulate collagen-making processes, or turn them off. Are we choosing to turn hydration genes on or off by our lifestyle choices? What about the genes that break down our collagen; is our diet inadvertently accelerating this process and leading to premature wrinkling? Or can we alter our diets to slow this process down and preserve our skin-plumping collagen?

The new science of what turns genes on and off is called epigenetics, which I will explain in more detail in Chapter Two. Epigenetics opens up a whole new perspective on how to address many different conditions in the body, including aging. Epigenetics turns the old adage, "your genes are your destiny," on its head. YOUR diet and lifestyle choices can help determine your future!

Two Pathways: Extrinsic & Intrinsic Aging

In the flow chart below, I have charted the molecular basis of skin aging. These are the therapeutic targets of the diet and lifestyle changes that I will be discussing the rest of the book—real-life tangible things that can be modified in order to influence skin aging. With this information, you become the artist of your own face.

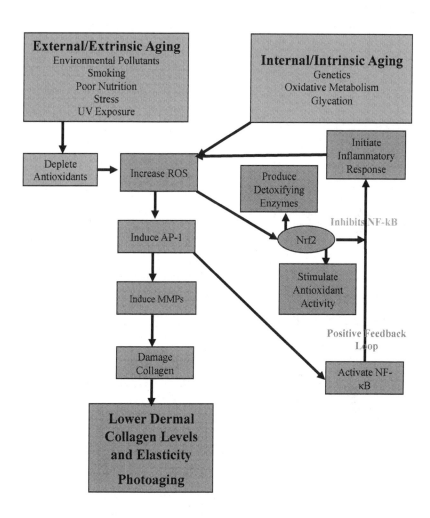

How Skin Ages Flow Chart

Deplete antioxidants refers to the fact that our skin contains a reservoir of antioxidants that inhibit the oxidation of other molecules (which leads to free radicals) in order to maintain skin health. Certain external/environmental triggers deplete these antioxidants, leading to our next step: **Increase ROS**.

Increase ROS refers to the Reactive Oxygen Species, otherwise known as free radicals, the highly reactive molecules that then proceed to form a chain reaction with other stable molecules, stealing electrons as they go, rendering the "attacked" molecule unstable and a free radical itself. This results in cell damage. Antioxidants fight free radicals; the depletion of antioxidants in the skin leads to an increase in free radicals and cellular damage resulting in premature skin aging.

Induce AP-1 is a transcription factor that turns genes on and off in response to a variety of external triggers. In the skin, it has multiple functions; but in this graphic it refers to the **induction of MMPs**, the next step in our flow chart. Simultaneously, AP-1 triggers the **activation of NF-kB**.

Induce MMPs Matrix Metalloproteinases, or MMPs, are the enzymes responsible for breaking down our collagen and elastin, which leads to wrinkles and sagging.

Activation of NF-kB means activating a transcription factor that turns on inflammation. In this diagram, we see that this inflammation is a positive feedback loop that generates even more reactive oxygen species (free radicals), which starts the whole wrinkle-producing cascade over again.

Damage Collagen is the result of this chain of events.

Photoaging is the scientific term for wrinkling and sagging that originates with UV damage from the sun.

Nrf-2 is a ray of hope in the midst of bad players. Nrf-2 represses multiple pro-inflammatory genes and regulates more than 200 genes critical for stimulating our own cellular production of antioxidants and detoxifying enzymes necessary for the metabolism of drugs and toxins. Yes, our bodies can make our own antioxidants, and I will reveal which plant foods enhance this production. Importantly, Nrf-2 also downregulates NF-kB.

Before we delve into the natural and healthy choices we can make for truly beautiful skin, let's look at the processes that actually cause skin aging. There are two main pathways to skin aging: the extrinsic (outside the body) pathway and the intrinsic (inside the body) pathway. Both can be positively influenced by making certain changes to diet and lifestyle resulting in YOU being the person who looks younger than your chronological age.

Extrinsic aging looks like:

- Deep wrinkles
- Age spots or hyperpigmentation
- Leathery skin

Intrinsic aging looks like:

- Fine wrinkles
- Thin and transparent skin
- Loss of underlying fat, leading to hollowed cheeks and eye sockets as well as noticeable loss of firmness on the hands and neck

- Bones shrink away from the skin due to bone loss, which causes sagging skin
- Dry skin that may itch
- Inability to sweat sufficiently to cool the skin
- Graying hair that eventually turns white
- Hair loss
- Unwanted hair
- Nail plates thin, the half-moons disappear, and ridges develops

Extrinsic Aging

Let's begin with extrinsic aging. Extrinsic means it comes from outside the body, so it includes processes like UV damage from the sun (consisting of UVA and UVB rays) and environmental factors such as pollution, smoking, poor nutrition, and stress. Extrinsic aging contributes about 85% of the skin aging load. These are all factors that we can control to an extent and therefore are amenable to interventions that can ameliorate their inexorable push towards skin aging.

> **Extrinsic Aging**
> - UV rays from sun
> - Pollution
> - Smoking
> - Poor Nutrition and Stress

A prime example of the idea of using an intervention to modify skin aging is using sunscreen to prevent not only sunburn and skin cancer, but also premature aging of the skin. Many studies have shown that UV rays are responsible for most (about 80%) of skin aging. This process is so well known that this type of aging has its own name: photoaging. Just look at a part of your body that never sees the sun, such as your butt, and compare it to your arms or face. The difference in skin quality is probably striking.

Until recently, no one had quantified just how much a daily sunscreen would delay aging. In recent news, a study published in the Annals of Internal Medicine in 2013, demonstrated that the group of people in the study (who lived in Australia and were under age 55) who applied sunscreen daily showed 24% less skin aging in four years than the group who simply applied sunscreen on a voluntary basis (for example, if they were going to go the beach that day). That's a phenomenal result in skin-age delay brought on by just one powerful change—the use of a daily sunscreen. With one easy step—the daily or morning application of sunscreen before you leave the house—you can look forward to 24% less skin aging in only four years. If you apply sunscreen daily for longer than four years, you are likely to gain even greater benefits.

Let's explore this concept in more depth. The sun produces both UVA and UVB rays, but UVA radiation is the biggest culprit in extrinsically accelerating the skin-aging process. This is because UVA radiation has the ability to penetrate more deeply into the dermis, which is beneath the epidermis, where it causes a gigantic explosion of Matrix Metalloproteinases (MMPs), enzymes that cut your collagen to pieces, while collagen production grinds to a halt. At the same time, free-radical formation skyrockets because the sun's rays deplete the reservoir of antioxidants naturally found in your skin that would otherwise combat free radicals.

Ironically, UVA radiation is not the type that causes sunburn. UVB radiation is the culprit behind sunburn. For decades, sunscreens have catered to this fact by only supplying a SPF rating based on the product's ability to absorb or deflect UVB rays. While applying a high enough SPF-rated sunscreen, for decades, people were able to spend more time in the sun without having to worry about getting sunburned. But, they had no idea that they were still aging their skin because UVA rays were **not** being blocked!

Nowadays, the damaging power of UVA rays are known, and sunscreens have begun to formulate based on preventing the damage of both kinds of sunlight. Be sure to look for this the next time you shop for a sunscreen or sunblock. You want a product that is designed to block both UVA and UVB radiation. These are readily available today and I highly recommend using them daily on your face. I will talk more about how to choose a good sunscreen later in the book.

Pollution as a whole, not just smoking, is now known to cause premature aging of the skin. The skin is our greatest barrier and protection against direct contact with various air pollutants. Recent studies have found that airborne particulate matter from air pollution results in premature skin aging in the form of age spots and wrinkling. Furthermore, the particles serve as carriers of other chemicals and metals that are capable of lodging in skin and promoting skin aging through free-radical damage. In a stunning discovery, certain phytochemicals in plant foods can actually turn down this cellular, gene-driven process! We will also discuss more direct methods of preventing pollution-stimulated, premature aging of the skin further in the book.

Smoking causes premature, extrinsic skin aging because nicotine narrows the blood vessels that serve your skin, thus reducing the amount of oxygen and nutrients that can reach your skin. This happens all over your body, not just on your face. According the American Lung Association, there are over 600 ingredients in a cigarette and, when burned, over 7000 chemicals are formed; 69 of these chemicals are known to cause cancer. So, smoking just adds to the overall pollution load of your body in addition to restricting oxygen and nutrient flow to the skin and producing an extraordinary amount of free radicals in the process.

Stress impacts skin too. Research has shown that skin is both an immediate stress perceiver and a target of stress responses. This we know intuitively from previous experiences with acne breakouts right before a big date or presentation, or a worsening of other skin conditions. Blushing is more evidence of the connection between our brain and our skin. I will devote an entire chapter to the damaging effects of stress on skin.

Dietary interventions designed for healthy aging have become a hot topic in nutritional epigenomic research as evidence continues to accumulate for nutritional factors influencing the aging process. In terms of skin health and beauty, nutritional strategies have shown promising results promoting overall health and vitality, which are reflected externally in more youthful-looking skin. Dietary interventions can improve skin health and beauty by quenching free radicals, dampening inflammation and glycation, all major players in the skin aging process.

Intrinsic Aging

Now let's move on to intrinsic aging, where metabolism and natural internal processes drive the aging process. Just by living, we are using an oxidative metabolism (we breathe oxygen) to run our physiological processes. Oxidative metabolism creates free radicals, which are considered to be one of the primary causes of aging. The aging effect of oxidation can be compared to how metal rusts when exposed to oxygen. We also experience a natural decline in hormones as we age, with noticeable effects on the skin. Another factor involved in intrinsic aging is glycation, or cross-linking, of proteins like collagen.

Oxidative Stress

Oxidative stress plays a major role in the skin-aging process. This is the common denominator between both intrinsic and extrinsic aging. Oxidative stress refers to the imbalance between damage-causing free radicals and the body's inherent ability to generate antioxidants to fight free radicals and produce enzymes to repair damaged DNA. Oxidative stress has been found to damage DNA, proteins, and lipids, which are the building blocks of our bodies. Oxidative damage is implicated in virtually every disease known to man, especially the chronic diseases of aging such as cardiovascular disease, Alzheimer's disease, Parkinson's disease, and cancer.

How does oxidative stress specifically contribute to skin aging? In intrinsic aging, large amounts of free radicals, which are present due to oxidative stress, activate collagen-eating enzymes, create inflammation, and then cascade down the same wrinkle-forming pathway as the extrinsic aging pathway. In other words, whether we are talking about extrinsic or intrinsic aging, we eventually find that they both lead to the wrinkle cascade depicted in Figure number one.

Antioxidants are compounds that fight or neutralize free radicals, thus putting an end to their DNA and cellular damage.

While some amount of free-radical formation is necessary and even desirable in our body under certain circumstances, excess free-radical formation has been found to overwhelm the body's own antioxidant defenses and result in aging and degenerative diseases associated with aging (more on how to increase antioxidant defenses later). Completely eradicating the production of free radicals in the body is not the goal here; indeed, studies have shown mixed results with the oral intake of antioxidants on various disease parameters.

Some environmental factors that increase free-radical formation in our bodies are environmental toxins, cigarette smoke, excessive sun exposure, and yes, even excessive exercise, due to the increased intake of oxygen and demands on the body. This is the reason why many long-distance runners and triathletes often look older than their age.

UV radiation and pollutants, such as polycyclic aromatic hydrocarbons found in car exhaust and air pollution, bombard the skin, producing free radicals on a daily basis. The skin is innately equipped to handle this barrage by having its own reservoir of antioxidants. In fact, skin is rich in antioxidants, mostly found in the epidermis, which bears the brunt of the resulting exposure-related oxidative damage. The problem is that this reservoir is quickly depleted upon exposure to these skin stressors, resulting in oxidative stress that damages the skin and is implicated in premature aging.

Later in this book, we will talk about how to not only increase your intake of these antioxidants that promote radiant skin through food and supplements, but also a secret way to stimulate your body's OWN production of antioxidants on a more consistent basis! There *is* a way to turn on your beauty genes, and this Master Switch gene is definitely one of the most important. Later, I will also present concrete steps that we can take to downregulate or suppress the damaging cellular processes related to oxidative stress and, thus, further decrease our rate of aging, leading to even more beautiful skin.

Glycation

Glycation is another newly discovered factor in skin aging that is a result of intrinsic forces. But outside forces, namely certain foods and cooking methods, can actually increase this process. While glycation occurs in our bodies naturally, excessive glycation has been associated with accelerated aging.

Glycation is a process where sugars attach to tissue proteins (such as collagen) to rearrange their youthful structure into something known as *advanced glycation endproducts* (AGEs). These aptly named AGEs damage collagen fibers and make them lose their elasticity and become rigid, more brittle, and prone to breakage, resulting in wrinkling, dryness, and looseness or crepiness in the skin. So these products called AGEs literally are AGING your entire body, including your skin.

It is known that diabetics exhibit the signs of aging sooner than non-diabetics. Part of this is due to the glycation process, which is demonstrated externally by premature aging of the skin. Of course, the glycation process is also occurring internally and wreaking havoc on various organs and blood vessels. In fact, the major blood marker used for monitoring blood sugar levels in diabetics is called hemoglobin A1c, which is nothing more than glycated hemoglobin (sugar-coated red blood cells).

A number of studies show that glycation of collagen increases not only with high levels of glucose, such as in diabetics, but also with normal levels of glucose over a very long time—that is, with age. This means glycation is a problem even in people who don't overconsume sugar. Once formed, AGEs induce cross-linking of collagen <u>even in the absence of glucose</u>. Glycation also induces cell death in skin cells. Furthermore, AGEs are accompanied by increased free-radical activity in skin collagen, a process that greatly accelerates skin aging. To make it worse, sun exposure facilitates glycation even further.

To add insult to injury, this intrinsic process kicks into gear around age 35 and then increases rapidly. The resulting AGEs are not reversible. A fascinating study published in 2013 examined the perceived age of older adults cross-referenced to their blood sugar level and discovered that, even in non-diabetics, the higher blood sugar participants were perceived to be older than their chronological age as compared to the participants with lower blood sugar levels. The perceived age of the diabetic group was even higher. The data showed that for each 1 mm/liter increase in blood sugar, the perceived age was increased by 5 months!

The formation of AGEs is now one of the hottest areas of research for understanding not only how the skin ages, but also for determining the mechanism of disease formation in the human body. In Chapter Three, we will see how you can dramatically decrease consumption of preformed AGEs in your diet simply by changing the way that you cook and knowing which foods are notorious sources of AGEs. Remember, prevention is key, as the process is irreversible.

Hormonal Imbalance and Decline

Hormones exert a tremendous effect on all parts of the body, including the skin. Part of the aging effect we see on women's skin is a result of the reduction of certain hormones in our bodies, like estrogen. During and after menopause, when estrogen levels decline, skin becomes thinner, more wrinkled, and drier. This is because estrogen stimulates collagen, which plumps up the skin and oils within the skin, which hold in moisture. Once moisture leaves, dry, flaky, and itchy skin can result.

Even before menopause, hormonal imbalances can plague the skin of anybody from puberty-on-up. Hormonal imbalances and deficiencies can be easily addressed through proper assessment and evaluation by your naturopathic physician or other integrative healthcare provider.

Pay particular attention to Chapter Nine on **Clean Products for Beauty** to learn which ingredients in your favorite skin-care and personal-care products may be endocrine disruptors—possibly the very culprits in your hormonal imbalance.

Where Extrinsic and Intrinsic Aging Meet

Both intrinsic and extrinsic aging lead to skin-aging and wrinkle formation, beginning with the degradation of antioxidants. Once the reservoir of antioxidants is depleted, free radicals are created that induce both oxidative stress and inflammation. The very process of inflammation further creates even more free radicals that feed forward into more inflammation, which just fuels the flames of the next steps of wrinkle formation: the degradation of collagen and resulting wrinkles.

Inflammation

It is now known that chronic inflammation is largely responsible for most of the chronic diseases of aging, including skin aging. Chronic, low-level inflammation that is not symptomatic (silent) is becoming known as "inflammaging," and inflammaging is a prime culprit in premature aging. Diet and lifestyle interventions designed for healthy aging have become a hot topic in nutritional epigenomic research. Patients are guided to make choices that guide their genes to turn on their health and vitality-promoting activities, and reduce inflammatory and health-destroying processes.

Silent inflammaging may not manifest on the skin with redness or rashes, but will provoke an insidious attack at the dermal levels of collagen and elastin fibers, the very substances that provide springiness and volume to our skin. This breakdown of collagen and elastin and slowdown of new collagen formation, along with the production of free radicals that further escalates the inflammatory cascade, results in wrinkles, loss of elasticity, pigment and texture changes that are the hallmarks of aging skin.

We will see later in the book concrete steps we can take to downregulate these cellular processes and thus decrease our rate of aging.

In the chapters ahead, you will find the secrets to and the science behind:

- How to turn down the genes responsible for prematurely aging your skin
- What to eat for younger-looking skin
- The secret "Master Switch" for turning on your youth-promoting genes
- What supplements to take for glowing skin
- How certain ingredients in your skin-care products are toxic and affecting your health and potentially the health of your future children
- How detoxification can literally clear the way for beautiful and radiant skin
- The intriguing link between gut health and skin health, and how to use this information to obtain radiant skin
- How stress and lack of beauty sleep are ruining your complexion

The main drivers of skin aging are environmental factors (such as solar radiation and pollution) and our own internal metabolism. These trigger the depletion of our antioxidant system, the creation of free radicals, increases in the enzymes that eat up our collagen, and result in inflammation leading to wrinkles. Fortunately, Mother Nature has provided solutions to these aging accelerators in terms of natural, powerful antioxidants and anti-inflammatories. The insights in this book are based on the latest scientific studies about skin aging that drill down to the molecular level. Use vanity as a leverage to modify your diet and lifestyle, not only to become more beautiful and radiant, but also to lower risks for the chronic diseases of aging. Restore your vitality and enthusiasm for life.

CHAPTER TWO

The New Science of Epigenetics and What That Means for Your Skin

If you are not science inclined, you may skip this section and move right into the more practical applications of this information.

EPIGENETICS IS AN EXCITING NEW FIELD that studies how our environment—much of which we can control—affects how DNA (our genes) expresses itself (or not) in our bodies. This means that environmental factors control the degree to which one might experience a disease, or whether or not one gets the disease at all. In terms of skin health, epigenetics represents a relatively unexplored territory that may well yield valuable clues in the way the future of skin care develops. By looking at methylation rates (one important epigenetic change) at key points on genes taken from skin cells, we already know that UVB-exposed skin is epigenetically different from non-exposed skin. In this book, we will see how our environment, from the food and nutritional supplements we ingest, to our thoughts and emotions, to our body burden of environmental toxins, influences the health and beauty of our skin.

"Epi" (Greek: over or above) literally means above, so epigenetics are the outside factors that influence DNA from "above." Yes, that's right; I said **influence**. Gone is the old construct of frozen-in-stone DNA, locked forever in a hopeless pattern of inevitability. Science is now reporting the secrets of how a serviceable portion of the human genome can be manipulated as we desire or pushed in an undesirable way unintentionally through our diet, lifestyle, thoughts, emotions, and environmental toxins.

Outside influences can have a **profound effect** on our genome (the sum of our genes), or our genetic "computer hardware." But computers can't operate without software; so, astonishingly, epigeneticists are studying how the epigenome, or "software instructions," tell the DNA to either produce the proteins that fuel our well-tuned physiology or **not** produce them. This is also known as turning genes on and off. Yes, using the analogy of a light switch, genes can be turned off and on, and many of these changes are reversible.

The epigenome is awake, alive, and responsive to environmental signals, especially during fetal development, but also throughout life. Many changes in gene expression persist long after toxic exposure has stopped. Among other things, this means that these changes can and do transcend generations.

When a gene has been turned on, it generates the one, very specific protein it was designed for. It is either doing it or it is not. If our goal is to avoid cancer, then our goal is to turn on (or keep on) the tumor-suppressor genes and turn off oncogenes (which can promote a cancer). So, we do have underlying genetic pre-dispositions; but, if we attempt to temper this with a healthy lifestyle, we increase the odds that we may never turn those oncogenes on while at the same time encouraging the active protein production of the tumor-suppressor genes.

Software cannot exist without someone to write it. Likewise, we can be the authors of much of our own, personal epigenome. What is the story you want to be told of your life? One of a joyous, vibrant, radiant person exuding passion and purpose, or one of illness, doctors, and pharmaceuticals? I'm exaggerating here to characterize my point: how, when, and if various pieces of our DNA are fired off or not depend to a large degree upon the decisions we make. To a very large degree, our health—*even at the genetic level*—is really up to us. We make at least one hundred different choices every day that either promote health or detract from it. These multiple choice-points throughout our day include our dietary choices, how we choose to move our body, what thoughts we choose to think, all the way to what time we choose to go to bed.

Our body is constantly reacting to our environment. The point is that what surrounds us, affects us. Likewise, the trillions of cells that make up each one of us swim in a continuous bath of changing environmental conditions. Our cells are quite responsive to this continuous onslaught of stimulus and, indeed, so are our DNA.

"It is becoming clear that a wide variety of common illnesses, behaviors, and other health conditions may have at least a partial epigenetic etiology, including cancer, respiratory, cardiovascular, reproductive, and autoimmune diseases, neurological disorders such as Parkinson's, Alzheimer's, and other cognitive dysfunctions, psychiatric illnesses, obesity and diabetes, infertility and sexual dysfunction. Effectors of epigenetic changes include many agents, such as heavy metals, pesticides, tobacco smoke, polycyclic

aromatic hydrocarbons, hormones, radioactivity, viruses, bacteria, basic nutrients, and the social environment, including maternal care. It has even been suggested that our thoughts and emotions can induce epigenetic changes."

- University of Pittsburgh researchers, Medical Hypotheses, 2009

Wow! This is a revolutionary statement, but it aligns magnificently with my own thinking on the nature of environment and health. This is exactly why I left my career in corporate finance to go back to naturopathic medical school many years ago.

Even the august *Time* magazine had a cover on epigenetics on January 19, 2010: "Why Your DNA Isn't Your Destiny: The new science of epigenetics reveals how the choices you make can change your genes – and those of your kids"

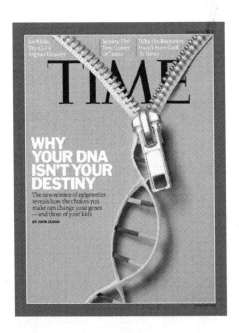

While modern healthcare has made enormous strides in emergency and trauma care, and infectious-disease control, most of modern-day illnesses are chronic in nature, according to the CDC. Our lifestyles have changed drastically over the last 100 years, and yet 100 years is not nearly long enough for our DNA to change appreciably in adaptation to our environment. These lifestyle changes include dietary changes from organic foods to foods that carry multiple pesticide, herbicide, and fungicide residues (before the 1940s, all food was organic because pesticides and herbicides had not been invented yet), unprocessed foods to processed, high mineral soils to low, yielding lower nutrient-dense foods and mineral-poor and pro-inflammatory diets. It is interesting to note that the same three, known DNA modifiers—poor nutrition, ever-increasing stress levels, and exposure to environmental toxins—are also linked to increasing incidences of cancer, obesity, type 2 diabetes, auto-immune diseases, and all chronic diseases in Westernized countries.

Epigenetics also has a darker side in that certain exposures in the womb have the ability to epigenetically modify germline (the egg and sperm) cells in the developing fetus, which can be passed down through the generations. It turns out that the developing fetus has several extremely vulnerable windows of time that are excruciatingly sensitive to environmental cues, and can result in illnesses that may not show up in the person until years or even decades later, or even in subsequent generations.

Nutritional status across the lifetime is now recognized as an important modulator of human health and chronic-disease risk. These complex relationships derive from studies on plasticity in developmental biology that are traceable to environmental effects. Food is comprised of bioactive compounds that influence epigenetic profiles by altering DNA methylation or histone modification, or by influencing the sufficiency or insufficiency of dietary substrates that are necessary for these enzymatic processes. What this really means is that food is information, or code, for our genome.

Nutritional-status influence is most important during pregnancy, as evidence from many studies suggest that nutritional experiences during critical periods of fetal development have epigenetic effects that persist throughout the life course. As one example, a recent study in rats found that a low-protein maternal diet during early pregnancy predisposed the offspring to type 2 diabetes due to epigenetic modification.

One of the largest natural, albeit tragic, experiments that demonstrates the effect of nutritional exposure on human development is the "Dutch Hunger Winter." During World War II the Dutch experienced a Nazi-induced famine during 1944-45 due to a blockade of food. This diet, which restricted calories to 400-800 calories per day even for pregnant women has yielded many research insights into the epigenetic effects of famine during pregnancy.

One of the most interesting observations from the Dutch Hunger Winter Study was that dietary deprivation of pregnant mothers that resulted in long-lasting consequences for adult health did not necessarily result in variations in birth weights. Women exposed to famine during the middle and late months of pregnancy did have babies with significantly reduced birth weights. However, babies born to mothers who were exposed to dietary deprivation only during early gestation (with the blockade ending prior to them giving birth) had normal birth weights due to intrauterine catch up growth. Yet, they still grew up to have higher rates of obesity than those born before and after the war, and those exposed to famine mid to late pregnancy.

A deprived fetal environment followed by an abundance of food in childhood may be a recipe for adult chronic disease. This is strikingly shown by comparing babies born to Dutch mothers during or shortly after the famine where food supplies were quickly replenished, and babies born during or shortly after the siege of Leningrad where food supplies were not so quickly replenished. In the case of the Leningrad babies who continued to have restricted nutrition and calories for a few years, no increase in obesity or cardiovascular disease was seen in adults. This suggests that intrauterine or infant/childhood catch up growth in times of abundance actually has a counterintuitive effect on health by promoting adult chronic diseases such as obesity and cardiovascular disease.

How Epigenetics Works

Epigenetic modifications consist mainly of DNA methylation, histone tail modification, and changes to microRNAs. The most studied of these modifications is DNA methylation, which means simply that a methyl group is attached to the gene. A methyl group can also be detached from the gene, so here is where the plasticity in gene expression comes in. They can be turned on and off. Often, when a gene is heavily methylated in a certain "promoter" region of the gene, that gene is silenced or turned off. It will not make a protein. If the gene is a tumor-suppressor gene, then turning it off is not desirable. If it is an oncogene, turning it off would be a smart move.

For example, a particular gene, GSTP1, is involved in making detoxification enzymes. Hyper-methylation, or too much methylation, has been shown to turn it off, meaning there is less detoxification capability to clear the body of toxicants that may be contributing to certain cancers. Green-tea polyphenols, on the other hand, have been shown to reactivate this gene by de-methylating it. Lycopene, a carotenoid, has been shown to do the same, at least in cell-culture studies. DNA methylation is very important in cancer development, as gene "silencing" of other well-known tumor-suppressor genes, such as P53 for example, can allow tumors to grow.

DNA strands are wrapped around histone proteins. One of the ways the epigenome is affected is by modifying the histones. When the histones are modified, it causes the DNA to either unwind (therefore becoming available for transcription or protein making) or wind up, making the DNA unavailable for transcription.

Help from Our Furry Friends

A striking example of the power of gene regulation, or epigenetics, is seen in agouti mice, in which genetically identical twins can look entirely different in both color and size. One mouse may be small and brown while its twin is yellow and obese. But DNA in each furry little mouse is identical, so how can this be? How can it be that the phenotype—or the way each mouse looks—is very different?

In the normal, healthy mouse, the agouti gene is kept in the "off" position because it has been methylated. But in the yellow and obese mice, the same gene has not been methylated, which means it has been turned "on" resulting in quite a different picture. Such obese mice (those with the gene in the "on" position), in addition to having a yellow coat instead of a brown one, are also more likely to suffer from diabetes and cancer as adults.

Mice with the agouti gene in the "off" position (caused by an epigenetic process of attaching methyl groups to DNA), have the gene for expressing black fur in the "on" position. This is the state of affairs for normal, healthy mice. But if the agouti gene is turned "on" thanks to a lack of methylation, the agouti protein binds to a melanin receptor located on a mouse's skin cells, which ends up blocking those cells from making black pigment. These are the unhealthy, obese mice that are hyperinsulinemic, more susceptible to cancer and, on average, live shorter lives.

Here's where it gets interesting. If you feed the pregnant mouse certain methyl donors, like folate and vitamin B12, the offspring are more likely to be born with the brown coat and be healthy because those methyl groups will methylate the gene in question. This is epigenetics in action—the environment (in this case, nutrition) affects the genome profoundly, either resulting in a healthy newborn mouse, or a mouse whose life will be prone to obesity, diabetes, and cancer.

One of the ways the agouti gene can become de-methylated (the agouti gene is turned on) is by exposure to the chemicals bisphenol A (BPA) and phthalates, ubiquitous compounds in our environment. Again, we see the production of yellow-coated, unhealthy offspring from mothers who were exposed to BPA and phthalates. On the other hand, supplementing the pregnant mice with methyl donors like folic acid or the phytoestrogen genistein improved upon this effect, even though the mothers were exposed to the BPA and phthalates.

This provides some phenomenal insight, both into the environmental toxicants that can cause deleterious health effects in offspring and into the protective effects of diet in the mother.

Shown below are the three main drivers of epigenetic influence. These can actually trigger gene expression (by producing the protein it was designed to produce) or silence the gene.

1) Diet/nutrition
2) Stress/emotions/thoughts
3) Environmental toxins

It is interesting to note that these same three known DNA modifiers have also been linked to increasing incidences of cancer, obesity, type 2 diabetes, autoimmune diseases, and other chronic diseases in Westernized countries. Naturopathic medicine already operates on the basis of using these environmental modifiers to get to the root of disease, and now we know why; these factors work through epigenetic means.

Diet/Nutrition

The Pima Peoples

Not far from my old Scottsdale office is a community of Pima Indians. They bear the horrific distinction of having the highest incidence of type 2 diabetes in the world. Thirty-eight percent of their population suffers from this debilitating disease. Compare this with an already shockingly high rate among all Americans of 8.3 percent. How is it then, that only 6.9 percent of the Pima of Mexico have this disease, despite having a *virtually identical genetic makeup* as the Arizonans?

The Pimas of Arizona live the average American lifestyle of processed foods, stress, and a lot of sitting. On the other hand, the Pimas of Mexico still live their native, active lifestyle of farming and eat the same way they did hundreds of years ago. As the Arizona Pimas generally drink Coca-Cola, eat processed food, and are not physically active, the Pimas of Mexico eat whole foods (see below) and physical activity is their way of life.

A 2006 study of the Pimas in both countries concluded that the much lower prevalence of type 2 diabetes and obesity in the Pima Indians in Mexico than in the United States indicates that, even in populations that are genetically susceptible to these problems, diet and lifestyle determine whether or not these genetic predispositions become reality. This study provides compelling evidence that lifestyle plays a major and underappreciated role in the global epidemic of type 2 diabetes and obesity.

Since this study was published, many more studies have followed that demonstrate epigenetic changes resulting in diabetes from chemicals in our environment, diet, and exercise.

The Pima Indians of Mexico include the following items in their traditional diet:

- Cornmeal and mesquite flour
- Tepary and pinto beans

- Pinole
- Sunflower seeds
- Posole
- Spinach
- Tomato
- Fruit
- Pumpkin seeds
- Salmon
- Chia seeds
- Squash
- Rabbit
- Cholla buds
- Blue popcorn

As you can see, processed foods and Coca-Cola do not appear on the list.

The challenges posed by diabetes in the U.S. are before us, not because so many of us have underlying diabetes genes (we do), but because we are so very sedentary, eat a processed and nutritionally bankrupt diet, and are exposed to environmental toxicants that have solid links to diabetes. Many of us (80 percent) don't even get enough exercise. So this means that we are not even *walking* enough! Far too many of us sit all day for our jobs, eat a big, unhealthy dinner, then watch television. This is exactly what turns on the genes that fuel diabetes!

On the other hand, the lives of our ancestors, morning to night, were filled with activity. Everything had to be done by hand and they had to walk everywhere. No modern conveniences were to be had. They were lucky if they got to sit down an hour or two each day! It is no wonder that the Institute of Medicine of the National Academies now recommends (finally) that we need a minimum of one hour a day of exercise.

Sitting is worse than smoking

Sitting has recently been shown to be more deadly than smoking. The number of hours we sit in a day has a **direct correlation** to how long we will live. As well, it is associated with all-cause mortality. This means that whatever will end up killing you in the end, a lifestyle of sitting will bring it on that much sooner. There is a clear and positive association between physical activity—before and after a major illness—and a longer life. The more hours active, the longer the life; period.

Some people have instituted a walking office. You walk on a treadmill with a good-sized desk in front of you. The machine's speed is set very low so you can actually do your work while you walk. What if many of us committed to just a few hours of such walking each day, how would our lives change? Quite a bit! We would feel more energy as our mitochondria become more active, gain muscle, lose weight, the rate of heart disease would go down, mental functioning would go up, and we would feel happier. Yes, simple exercise really does all that.

I was recently introduced to another alternative desk structure in an office, and that was a standing desk. There is no treadmill involved, just a desk situated at a higher height than a regular desk, and no chair. This pretty much solves the sitting problem. And then I have also seen the standing conference table. This is very clever because, while you are standing up at your meeting, you are very motivated to be productive and get the meeting over with, so that you can go back to your desk and sit down.

Breaking up the day with walking and other forms of exercise is vitally important to counteract the insidious effects of sitting all day. Many doctors will recommend a five- or ten-minute break every hour where stretching and light activity is encouraged. I invite you to find what works best for you, but you must move.

Stress/Emotions/Thoughts/Beliefs

The mind-body connection is certainly not a new concept. Mind-body medicine uses the power of thoughts and emotions to influence physical health. As Hippocrates once wrote, "The natural healing force within each one of us is the greatest force in getting well." Do you hear that? We all have a doctor within! And this doctor is on call 24-7, with never a wait, no pesky insurance forms to fill out, and has complete focus on you.

In nearly every single medical model in the world, besides Western medicine, the emphasis is on the mind influencing the body. In Western medicine, however, the mind and the body have been separated completely and all emphasis is on the body part that seems to be having the problem. This body part is viewed as an isolated cog in a complex machine that simply needs the right technician (specialist) to make an adjustment, and then the cog is fixed and the machine will run properly again.

In reality, our minds are pretty much running the whole show. The mind and body are intrinsically and dynamically coupled. Perceptions, thoughts, and feelings change, and reciprocally respond to, the state of the body.

I remember reading a pivotal book while I was in medical school in the 1990s called Molecules of Emotion by Candace Pert, PhD. The author, at one time, was the chief of brain chemistry at the National Institutes of Health who went on to discover that emotions were brokered by neuropeptides (emotions had biochemistry behind them), which had receptors all over the body including on the immune, endocrine, muscular, and skeletal systems, not just on the neurological system. She demonstrated, for the first time, that the mind was in the body and vice versa.

This is why our emotions, our thoughts, and feelings can affect our bodies. For example, stressed-out students have been shown in numerous clinical trials to get sick right after a stressful event such as final exams. In fact, stress is well known to make just about any physical ailment worse.

Skin cells also have receptors for neurotransmitters. In fact, the nervous system and our skin derive embryonically from the same cells: the ectoderm. This is why emotions can and do show up on our skin. The basic blush, for example, shouts to the world that you are embarrassed. The dreaded pimple before a first date also clues us in that stress can affect our skin.

Researchers have begun to study these emotional connections to skin with some surprising and interesting results. In one study of elderly adults with atopic dermatitis, viewing a funny movie for two hours increased their testosterone levels in their saliva while reducing their trans-epidermal water loss (TEWL) as compared to the control group of elderly adults with healthy skin. In the elderly population, dry skin can be a problem—and a reduction in TEWL means less dry skin.

A very recent article published in the journal *Beneficial Microbes* titled "Acne vulgaris: probiotics and the gut-brain-skin axis: from anecdote to translational medicine", brings us back to the inherent holism found in our bodies. This article reviewed the gut-brain-skin axis and contemplates not only the effects of emotions on skin, but the overlapping effect of emotions on our gut microbes, which also affects the skin. The article builds on a couple of prescient dermatologists from the 1930s, John Stokes and Donald Pillsbury, who postulated that emotional states such as depression and anxiety could alter normal intestinal flora, which increased intestinal permeability, resulting in inflammation manifesting on the skin as acne. Eighty years later, this hypothesis has enjoyed a resurgence and the study of intestinal flora, psychological stress, and skin is being explored with an eye towards greater understanding and treatment options for multiple skin diseases, not just acne. The gut microbiota, or microbiome, is one of the hottest research areas today due to its profound influence on the entire body.

Environmental Toxins

One of the largest classes of epigenetic triggers is that of environmental toxins. There is now mounting evidence that exposures to environmental toxins, particularly in early fetal or neonatal development, can induce epigenetic changes which may be transmitted into **subsequent generations** and/or serve as the basis for developing diseases in later life.

In one recent study published in the Proceedings of the National Academy of Sciences in 2012, it was found that a single exposure of a commonly used fungicide to pregnant rats, resulted in *three* generations of altered stress responses in the offspring. The subsequent generations were **not exposed to the fungicide at all!** The fungicide in question, vinclozolin, is used on vineyards, fruits and vegetables, and even golf courses. The unanticipated epigenetic effect of additives, including pesticides and fungicides, on current and future generation's health is one good reason for eating organic food whenever possible.

At the same time, there is evidence that certain *diet and lifestyle changes can change back some previously created, environmentally-induced changes.* Remember, epigenetic changes are usually transient and reversible; there is no change to the underlying DNA, otherwise it would be called a gene mutation. This is also why certain positive lifestyle changes must be incorporated consistently, otherwise the positive changes will not maintain. At the same time, it may be possible to overcome previously unhealthy manifestations in our bodies with a change to more healthful strategies. As the study of epigenetics is still new, this is one area I imagine will receive quite a bit of research and attention.

How we decide to live our lives actually affects gene expression. For example, does cancer run in your family? Cancer rates are expected to continue to increase such that one in three women and one in two men will get cancer in their lifetime, according to the National Cancer Institute. This has increased dramatically over the last few decades and clearly reveals that environmental forces are at play, since our genes have not changed. What that means is we all need to be cognizant that more than family history and genetics are involved in cancer, and that we all need to take heed of diet and lifestyle factors that can help us prevent cancer.

Today, one of the more exciting research focuses is the use of food as cancer preventive agents. There are foods and spices that have been shown to be epigenetically active against cancer. As epigenetic changes have been found to be involved at the earliest points in tumor development, food as medicine has become an attractive target for cancer prevention. Clinical trials are underway to explore the epigenetically active role of foods in cancer. Not surprisingly, many phytochemicals present in plant foods, particularly the flavonoids, are suggested to be able to alter epigenetic cellular mechanisms.

Foods That Affect Epigenetics Involved in Cancer

- Green-tea polyphenols
- Soy isoflavones
- Apple/Coffee polyphenols
- Black raspberries
- Curcumin
- Selenium
- Isothiocyanate (from cruciferous vegetables)
- Vitamin A
- Lycopene (from tomatoes)

Gerhauser C. Cancer Chemoprevention and Nutri-epigenetics: State of the Art and Future Challenges *Top Curr Chem* 2012

This is where the magic is! Unlike that so-last-century idea of "set in granite" genes, the new model of epigenetics sings to us in glorious, celebratory verse that there is an exquisite, dynamic interaction between our genes and our environment. We are not passive pawns in this extraordinary communication; rather, if we choose, we can be enthusiastic participants.

CHAPTER THREE

Eating for Beauty

"Food is what actually feeds, repairs, and rejuvenates your skin cells."—Dr. Fine

IN THIS CHAPTER, WE WILL COVER why some foods are good for beauty and health, and some are bad. We will also discuss how to turn on your own Master Switch, which turns on your body to make its own antioxidant and detoxifying genes—a super shortcut to better health and beauty.

Diet is one of the most powerful epigenetic factors that influences your skin quality and how well you age. It does this by modifying the fundamental processes at the cellular and genetic levels that are responsible for aging, such as the genes that affect collagen (which gives skin its structure and strength) or inflammation (which leads to skin wrinkling). Epigenetics through nutrition, or nutriepigenomics, is an attractive tool to support healthy gene optimization in the aging process.

The father of medicine himself, Hippocrates, proclaimed: "Let food be thy medicine and medicine be thy food."

Your skin also reflects your inner health; when you are healthy on the inside, your skin glows, is blemish free, and has even skin tone, texture, and fewer lines. The connection between gut health and skin, although not well known, has a profound effect on your skin.

Some recent key findings from epigenetic research look at differences in how genes are expressed in older and younger skin, and how certain foods may affect these genes. For example, in Chapter Two on Epigenetics, we saw that the type of diet fed to pregnant mice affected the hair color of the offspring permanently—even for all future generations. This was a remarkable demonstration of how certain genes are turned on or off, depending on what was eaten.

In addition, several aging studies of identical twins have been performed that illustrate the effect different environmental influences have on facial skin aging. The fact is, even genetically identical twins age at different rates. Truly, aging represents a fundamental epigenetic phenomenon due to the high degree of influence found in the environment.

The main drivers of skin aging, caused either by environmental factors such as solar radiation or our own metabolism, are depletion of our antioxidant system, creation of free radicals, increases in the enzymes that break down collagen (MMPs), glycation, and inflammation. Fortunately, nature has provided solutions to these aging accelerators.

The Solutions

Antioxidants

Antioxidants are necessary for anti-aging because they, by definition, mop up the reactive oxygen species, or free radicals, generated by intrinsic and extrinsic aging processes. For this reason, antioxidants are a first-line defense against aging. One of the reasons fruits and vegetables are so important in a healthy diet is that they are chock full of antioxidants. One special group of antioxidants, polyphenols—naturally occurring chemicals derived from plants, fruits, nuts, vegetables, and teas—have received the most attention because they have been proven to have many beneficial health benefits. They are also widely abundant and relatively inexpensive making them attractive targets to reseachers for a cost-effective alternative to current pharmacologic therapeutics. So why not just eat them as part of a varied, whole-food, plant-based diet? Or better yet, juice them?

I highly recommend getting a varied antioxidant portfolio from eating a wide variety of plant foods. Taking individual antioxidants in supplemental form, in high doses, can actually have a pro-oxidant effect, instead of an antioxidant effect. Part of the problem is that antioxidants work together; they have synergistic effects. By supplementing with high doses of one, you throw off this synergy. By consuming your complement of antioxidants through eating many different servings of colorful fruits and vegetables each day, you are not overconsuming one antioxidant over another.

Having seven to nine servings of organic produce each day provides a rich array of antioxidants, vitamins, and minerals, and a huge class of phytonutrients for the body. Does that sound overwhelming? Most people struggle to get one fruit and one vegetable into their diet each day. One way to ingest a lot of servings of produce at once is to juice. I am personally a big juicing fan, and started in my early twenties. Juicing is an easy and delicious way to start the day, requires no digestion, provides an abundance of energy with no caffeine, and paves the way for great aging on the inside and out, while nourishing the body at a cellular level. At the end of this chapter, I will provide my personal recipe for juicing; it is great for skin aging and factors in much of what we will talk about in this chapter.

Studies have shown that it is, in fact, possible to delay skin aging and improve skin conditions through the use of antioxidants. The most important source of antioxidants is provided through sound nutritional choices. The most well-known systemic antioxidants shown to be beneficial in the skin are vitamins C, E, the carotenoids, and the trace elements copper and selenium. Vitamin C is absolutely

crucial for collagen formation.

Feed Your Skin These Antioxidant-Rich Foods

- Apples
- Asparagus
- Avocado
- Beets
- Blackberries, blueberries, raspberries, strawberries
- Cherries
- Broccoli
- Chocolate/cocoa
- Ginger

- Green tea
- Kale, spinach, and other dark leafy greens
- Olive oil
- Parsley
- Pears
- Plums
- Pomegranate

One of the inherent problems in antioxidants, either consumed in foods or supplements, is their very short half-lives. That means even an hour after you take in antioxidants, they may be gone, metabolized, used up. This is why it is so important to consume a diet rich in antioxidants throughout the day.

However, we also have a way to counteract all these free radicals on our skin that works from the inside out. Our cells have the amazing ability to make their own antioxidants and detoxifying enzymes. Recently, the discovery of Nrf-2, aka **The Master Switch,** a transcription factor that turns on certain activities of a cell, has energized the scientific community. Nrf-2 is known as the "master regulator" of cellular antioxidant defenses. When the Nrf-2 system is turned on, your cells will produce their own antioxidants and detoxifying enzymes on a more continuous basis. This is profound— that we have the ability to make our own antioxidants and detoxifying elements. The trick is to know which foods, spices, and other environmental factors turn on Nrf-2. This is one of the most exciting recent developments in health; our ability to stimulate this system at will.

More specifically, how can Nrf-2 stimulation help our skin? Nrf-2 activation provides the skin protection against BOTH Ultraviolet A and B radiation, which, as we've seen, are oxidizing agents "that cause significant damage to cellular components that leads to photoaging and cancer." This is because Nrf-2 performs two important functions: it protects the skin from harmful UV rays by producing antioxidants and quenching free radicals, and also detoxifies the skin.

The skin is the largest organ in the body. It provides the first line of defense to the body against damage from environmental factors. When the skin is damaged by means of a wound, Nrf-2 activation is upregulated, or enhanced, in the area of the wound. This helps the skin and body protect themselves and promotes recovery. The formulation of Nrf-2 topical products for the skin has already begun; but what I propose is better: Nrf-2 activation from within so that your skin and your organs both benefit. After all, you are aging on the inside too.

Foods and Spices That Turn On Nrf-2

- Green tea
- Broccoli and other cruciferous vegetables
- Ginger
- Garlic
- Curcumin
- Olive oil
- Fish oil
- Lycopene (tomatoes, red/pink grapefruit, watermelon, papaya, mango)

So how can we use diet to epigenetically modify those genes responsible for skin aging?

The most powerful strategy we can undertake to achieve beauty is to eat for beauty. And since we eat about three times per day, we have ample opportunity to practice good nutritional skin care. You really are what you eat. **Food is information for your genes**, it tells them what to turn on and what to turn off. Below, I will go into detail about the benefits of specific foods that are excellent for repairing and maintaining your skin health and radiance.

Green Tea

Tea is the most widely consumed beverage in the world, after water. Many human and animal studies have shown that green-tea catechins, a subcategory of polyphenols, provide protection from the sun's UV rays. Green tea is also an antioxidant-rich item that promotes healthy, glowing skin through multiple mechanisms. Many published studies have shown that green tea's antioxidants, mainly epigallocatechin-3-gallate (EGCG), can help prevent UV-induced skin cancer. In fact, a large review published in 2012 in the Journal, *Oxidative Medicine and Cellular Longevity*, concluded that "Green tea is an abundant source of plant polyphenols that exhibit significant antioxidant, chemopreventive, and immunomodulatory effects in protecting the skin."

In the *Journal of Nutrition* (2011), researchers found that green-tea polyphenols provide photoprotection, increase microcirculation, and modulate the skin properties of women. In a 12-week, double blind, placebo-controlled study, 60 women were given either one liter of green tea providing 1402 total catechins per day, or one liter of a control beverage. At the end of 12 weeks, the women in the green-tea group experienced 25% less burning from UV light, and had improved skin-structural characteristics like elasticity, roughness, scaling, density, and water homeostasis. In a separate test, green tea was found to increase microcirculation 30 minutes after ingesting. Microcirculation is vastly important because it is blood flow that brings oxygen and nutrients to the skin; the blood feeds the skin. Improved elasticity is important, because loss of elasticity is why skin sags.

Green tea also protects DNA from damage caused by UV radiation. In several studies with mice, both orally consumed and topically applied green tea was shown to be protective against non-melanoma skin cancer. The green-tea polyphenols accomplished this through rapidly repairing the DNA breakage caused by the solar radiation.

This result was repeated in a study with human skin. Topical treatment with green-tea polyphenols 20 minutes before sun exposure decreased the amount of UVB induced DNA damage. Since this DNA damage is what leads to skin cancer, this data suggests that green-tea polyphenols may be a possible strategy to reduce the risk of skin cancer in the human population.

Green-tea polyphenols have also been shown to block the free radicals (ROS) produced by UV light and restore epidermal antioxidant enzymes. Remember, stopping the free radical damage mitigates the downstream damage on the aging chart.

Dermatologists are very interested in green-tea polyphenols because they have been shown to inhibit tumor invasion and angiogenesis, thereby preventing tumor growth and metastasis. Could green tea become a part of a preventive program for skin cancer?

From these findings, it can be seen that orally consumed EGCG has two different mechanisms of action and can act as both a chemopreventive and photochemopreventive drug; it can protect the body by suppressing, slowing down, and reversing the process of carcinogenesis, as well as protect the skin from damaging radiation caused by harmful UVB rays. This not only prevents photo-damage, but also premature aging of the skin and skin cancer.

Green tea is one of the best skin beautifiers available. Green-tea polyphenols have the ability to beautify and protect our skin by safeguarding our collagen.

Berries

Berries as a class enjoy a favored position as top anti-cancer, skin-beautifying, and antioxidant-rich foods. These little gems are packed full of powerful phytonutrients that feed your skin.

Blueberries are one of the superstar anti-inflammatory and antioxidant agents. These little jewels possess supercharged antioxidant and anti-inflammatory powers and are packed with phytonutrients called anthocyanins, which are the pigments responsible for their deep, dark, rich color. Scientific studies have revealed that anthocyanins naturally avert glycation-induced damage by stabilizing the collagen matrix, promoting collagen synthesis, and improving microcirculation. This was first discovered by studying the effects of bilberry (the European blueberry) on the formation of cataracts, a classic example of glycation-induced damage in the eye.

The effect of blueberries on skin aging is even more impressive, as they exert epigenetic effects on skin. In addition to blocking glycation, blueberries inhibit matrix metalloproteinases (MMPs), which are the enzymes responsible for breaking down collagen. MMPs increase with age and greatly contribute to skin wrinkling and aging. Blueberry polyphenols also are anti-inflammatory and downregulate the skin aging caused by skin inflammation.

Raspberries are another berry known for having many beneficial effects on the body. Ellagic acid, which is one of the polyphenols found in berries and which is particularly highly concentrated in raspberries, prevents the degradation of dermal elastic fibers while at the same time enhancing the formation of new elastin in the skin. This helps to prevent sagging. Ellagic acid also mediates inflammation, preventing wrinkling. At the same time, ellagic acid is known for its cancer prevention ability; a plus when considering that skin cancer is the most prevalent cancer in humans in the United States, according to the CDC (Centers for Disease Control).

In one study, ellagic acid was found to completely inhibit the breakdown of collagen induced by UVB radiation in human skin cells. This occurred through a blockade of the MMP enzymes that degrade the collagen in skin, resulting in skin wrinkles.

Pomegranate

Another skin-regenerating powerhouse is the pomegranate which, like the blueberry, also exerts its salutatory effect on the skin through epigenetics. Pomegranates are rich in phenolic compounds such as ellagic acid, punicalagin, and punicic acid. Topically, pomegranate extract promotes skin health in several ways: by increasing dermal skin cell proliferation and collagen synthesis, as well as inhibiting collagen-degrading MMPs, thus protecting against the aging effects of the sun and inflammation.

When taken internally, the juice, seeds, and even the peel confer anti-cancer, anti-inflammatory, and skin-saving properties. Recent research has shown that pomegranate extracts selectively inhibit the growth of breast, prostate, colon, and lung cancer cells in culture. In preclinical animal studies, oral consumption of pomegranate extract inhibited growth of lung, skin, colon, and prostate tumors. An initial phase II clinical trial of pomegranate juice in patients with prostate cancer reported significant prolongation of prostate specific antigen doubling time, which means that the cancer is not growing as quickly.

Pomegranate juice has been shown to be effective in ameliorating UV-mediated damage in human skin cells—the sun photoaging effect. So, if the UV damage is prevented, the cascade of inflammation (NFkB) and oxidative stress (decrease in ROS and Nrf-2 activation) is prevented, resulting in prevention of wrinkles. Pomegranate seems to have it all with respect to skin health: it wards off sun damage, reduces inflammation, helps produce collagen, fights free radicals with its own antioxidant arsenal, and then activates our own cellular machinery for ramping up our levels of antioxidants and detoxifying enzymes.

Pomegranate oil has been shown to actually regenerate the epidermis, or outer layer of skin, by stimulating keratinocytes (skin cells). This is due to its being a potent source of a Omega-5 conjugated fatty acid and beneficial phytoestrogen—a rare plant source of CLA (conjugated linoleic acid). CLAs are mostly found in animal foods such as beef and milk and much more so in grass fed cows. This study joins a growing body of research supporting pomegranate seed oil as a topical skin treatment. In another study of pomegranate seed oil, topical application was shown to significantly decrease the incidence of skin cancer in mice after exposure to carcinogenic chemicals. This is the reason I have included pomegranate seed oil in my own formulation called Youth Serum.

Cruciferous Vegetables

Sulphoraphane is another skin powerhouse. This phytonutrient found in cruciferous vegetables such as kale, bok choy, chard, and broccoli is a multifunctional wonder food. In terms of skin health, sulphoraphane epigenetically downregulates AP-1, collagen-wrecking MMPs, and inflammation-instigating NFkB, while at the same time epigenetically turning on Nrf-2, thereby stimulating the cellular mechanisms that generate antioxidants and also phase-2 detoxification enzymes, including glutathione. Naturally, sulphoraphane does this all over the body, not just on the skin, so it provides chemoprevention and inflammation fighting all over. This is one phytonutrient you want to make sure to include every day.

Intestinal flora, or the bacteria in the gut, greatly influences how a person ages, including on the skin. Studies have identified the Japanese as people who age gracefully and have some of the longest-living people on earth. Researchers have discovered that the traditional Japanese diet has a beneficial effect on their aging process. The Japanese consume ample amounts of green tea, root vegetables (especially cruciferous vegetables), and fish, which they prepare in a way that does not form AGE (Advanced Glycation Endproducts) products in the body. So their diet is already a low glycation diet, which reduces skin wrinkling.

Green tea and cruciferous vegetables actually promote good bacteria formation in our intestinal tracts. A popular spice used in

Japan, ginger, also promotes the growth of *Lactobacilli*, one of the beneficial gut bacteria species. The combination of a high-vegetable diet (high in both cruciferous vegetables and fiber), green tea, ginger, omega-3 fatty acids from fish, and lack of AGE-promoting food preparation, contributes to smoother and more youthful-looking skin in the Japanese.

Another aspect of sulphoraphane that deserves special mention is the fact that it induces phase-2 detoxification enzymes all over the body, including skin cells. Detoxification is an important and entirely overlooked contribution to skin aging, and will be discussed further in subsequent chapters.

Sulphoraphane is also a tyrosinase inhibitor, which means it inhibits melanin production and, hence, age spots. Truly, you will want to include these foods in your anti-aging food repertoire as there are not very many foods that also help with skin brightening.

Carotenoids

Vitamin A, a skin-beautifying vitamin that was discussed in Chapter Two, is a broad family of related antioxidant nutrients. Some vitamin A comes from animal foods. The plant sources of pre-vitamin A are grouped together in the carotenoid family. The carotenoids are then converted in the body to vitamin A. Vitamin A plays a key role in skin diseases and is known to help repair damaged tissues.

> **Existing Vitamin A sources:**
> * Beef and lamb liver
> * Eggs

- Butter
- Cod liver oil

Carotenoid sources:

- Sweet potato
- Carrot
- Spinach, kale, and other dark leafy greens
- Winter squash
- Cantaloupe

The carotenoid family contains the phytonutrients β-carotene, lutein, zeaxanthin, and lycopene, which also have skin-beautifying properties. Carotenoids are found in carrots, tomatoes, dark leafy greens, sweet potatoes, mangos, cantaloupe, pumpkin, and squash. β (beta)-carotene is found prominently in the skin and is a photoprotector. Its ability to prevent UV-induced skin damage has been demonstrated in various studies. The carotenoid family decreases reactive oxygen species, inhibits AP-1, thus downregulating the MMP pathway which destroys collagen and produces wrinkles. Carotenoids also downregulate NFkB, heading off damaging inflammation.

A fun fact about carotenoids is that these deeply pigmented fruits and vegetables actually cause a change in your own skin's color, producing a golden glow that a recent study revealed made those people more attractive to people of the opposite sex. So say yes to carrots! Who can resist a golden, naturally derived glow that you didn't have to sit out in the sun's photodamaging rays to obtain?

Lycopene, another carotenoid, deserves a special mention because it is an Nrf-2 stimulator—it turns on your own antioxidant machinery to fight wrinkle formation from free radicals. This is why lycopene is popping up in so many internal and topical anti-aging treatments. Lycopene is found in tomatoes, papaya, watermelon, and grapefruit; it is what gives these foods their red color.

Resveratrol, found in grapes, wine, chocolate, and peanuts, is a wonderful skin preserver as well. Resveratrol is known to be a potent antioxidant, downregulating AP-1, MMP, NFkB and, if that isn't enough, it too is a Nrf-2 stimulator. Resveratrol is spawning an entire industry relating to its many anti-aging and health-promoting effects in the body.

Fats

Did you know that skin is hydrated mostly from within the body? A moisturizer will plump up the skin by temporarily providing moisture from the outside, partly by blocking the evaporation of water from the skin. But proper hydration on the inside is necessary for skin to look hydrated and fresh. That means plenty of water. I recommend dividing your weight by two and drinking that amount of water, in ounces, per day. If you live in a desert or exercise frequently, more is needed.

In addition to water, the fats you eat make a difference on your skin. The fat you eat helps your skin hold onto moisture, smoothing and plumping the surface. Dietary fats are also important because they are incorporated into the cellular membranes, fortifying and making them flexible, helping to keep your skin supple, elastic, and youthful-looking. Contrary to what you might believe, a study published in the *American Journal of Clinical Nutrition* demonstrated that women with a higher intake of healthy fats had fewer wrinkles and firmer skin tone.

Another study compared types of fats and found that those who consumed the most olive oil had reduced facial aging. Yet a different study, this time on Japanese women, found that higher intakes of total fat, saturated fat, and monounsaturated fat, was significantly associated with increased skin elasticity. The same study also found that a higher intake of green and yellow vegetables was significantly associated with a decreased wrinkling score.

Fats also help you absorb protective antioxidants like vitamin E, beta-carotene, and lycopene. A study in the *Journal of Nutrition* found that adding avocado to a salad increased the absorption of these fat-soluble nutrients up to 15 times. You very much want these antioxidants because they will protect your skin against UV damage that contributes to skin aging and cancer.

The avocado is a nutritional superfood and antioxidant powerhouse, especially when it comes to skin health. Not only does it provide moisturization from the inside-out, but it also protects against UVB-induced damage and inflammation in the skin while enhancing DNA repair. These photo-protective efforts protect against both premature skin aging and skin cancer.

Did you know that half of an avocado contains 4.6 grams of fiber, 345 mg of potassium, 57 mg of phytosterols, 114 calories, and just 0.2 grams of sugar? That's a lot of skin-friendly nutrients and high-quality fats packed into a tasty and creamy food.

Bone Broth

I am sure you are familiar with collagen creams which claim to restore in your skin what time has taken away. After all, collagen decreases with age and it would seem like simply applying it to your skin would help. But the secret that the skin-care industry does not want you to know is that most of the collagen creams on the market do not penetrate your skin; the collagen molecule is simply too big. These products do not work, but they are always hailed as a skin-care miracle.

I have two words for a true skin-care miracle: bone broth. Bone broth is rich in gelatin derived from collagen released from the breakdown of bones and joints. Enjoying bone broth on a regular basis not only helps heals the gut, but nourishes the skin and your joints with orally consumed collagen that makes a beeline for your skin.

Fish and Fish Oil

Eating fish and fish oil also keeps the skin radiant, supple, and wrinkle-free. The omega-3 fatty acids found in fish, especially wild salmon and other cold-water fish, are anti-inflammatory, enhance elasticity, protect collagen, and limit UV-induced skin damage. Oily fish, such as salmon, sardines, anchovies, and mackerel, are very high in these skin-protecting, anti-inflammatory, omega-3 fatty acids called eicosapentaenoic acid (EPA) and docasahexaenoic acid (DHA).

EPA from fish oil has been shown to inhibit MMPs, the collagen-shredding enzymes and cause your skin to become aged and wrinkled. As collagen production slows as we age, it is extremely important to block these enzymes that break it down.

And what about loss of elasticity in the skin? A study in the *Journal of Dermatological Treatment* showed a 10% improvement in skin elasticity among women who consumed just over 1 gram of

EPA-rich fish oil for three months. This is not a very large dose of fish oil! However, the average intake of omega-3 derived EPA and DHA for Americans is only 100 mg per day, so the dose prescribed in the study is ten times the average American's consumption.

One of omega-3 fatty acid's chief characteristics is that it is a strong anti-inflammatory agent. In part, it achieves this through downregulation of one of the transcription factors for inflammation: NFkB (see skin aging flow chart in Chapter One). As inflammation is one of the driving factors of skin aging and wrinkling, it is easy to see how adding fish and fish oil to your diet would be a smart move.

In a bonus move, omega-3 fatty acids also stimulate the Nrf-2 intrinsic antioxidant manufacturing system. Revving up your body's own production of antioxidants provides even more free-radical-damage protection than ingesting antioxidants in supplemental form. And remember, free radicals at the top of the aging chart start the facial wrinkling cascade.

On the subject of fish contamination, most of the concern centers around the mercury content found in fish. How does mercury get into our fish? Mercury is released into the air from coal-fired power plants, the incineration of medical and municipal waste, and other industrial sources. Once in the air as air pollution, it travels around the globe on air currents and then drops back into the ocean, lakes, streams, and rivers, where it bio-accumulates up the food chain, into the fish, and then into you. The more fish you consume, the higher your levels of methylmercury. Mercury is a heavy metal known to have adverse effects on the nervous system, kidneys, reproductive system, and the developing fetus.

There are various guides on the internet to mercury levels found in various fish. Review these guides to determine which fish is safest and wisest for your needs. The website below is one such guide:

http://www.nrdc.org/health/effects/mercury/guide.asp

While fish is the most common source of methylmercury in humans, an underappreciated source of inorganic mercury poisoning in women is found in imported skin-lightening cosmetic products. Skin-lightening creams are some of the most popular cosmetic creams in the world, particularly in countries where skin tones are darker. Unfortunately, mercury is a good and cheap skin lightener and, while the FDA does not approve mercury for use in skin-care products in the United States, other countries have no such qualms.

So if you have imported skin-lightening creams, typically from the Middle East, Asia, or Latin America, look for the following terms on the list of ingredients: "mercurous chloride," "calomel," "mercuric," "mercurio," or "mercury" and, if you see it, stop using the product immediately. Occasionally, mercury is not even listed on the ingredients.

For those who do not wish to consume fish or fish oil, omega-3 fatty acids are also found in chia seeds, walnuts, flax seeds, hulled hemp seeds, and purslane, a green leafy vegetable. Vegetarian sources of omega-3s provide only ALA (alpha-linolenic acid), a precursor form that the body cannot convert as efficiently to the DHA and EPA that fish oil provides, but is still beneficial for the body.

Dietary Strategies

As far as actual diets or dietary strategies are concerned, the best diet for skin is an anti-inflammatory diet. This makes sense if we look at our skin-aging chart and see that inflammation is one of the main drivers of skin aging and wrinkling. Interestingly, the Mediterranean Diet has long been associated with healthy aging, and it is a good representation of an anti-inflammatory diet.

One of the biggest dietary factors causing inflammation is food allergies. I have found over my many years of testing patients for food allergies, that the vast majority of people have them. Testing for (and eliminating) food allergies is one of the cornerstones to good health and leads to healthy skin. However, food allergies are a symptom of a deeper problem in the gut which also has to be healed. Eliminating problematic foods is the start to healing the gut.

Food allergies lead to systemic inflammation in the body, which not only leads to puffiness in the face (and other parts of the body), but also wrinkles, skin rashes, and blemishes.

The top food allergies are:

- Gluten containing grains: wheat, rye, barley
- Dairy
- Eggs
- Soy
- Sugar (don't use sugar substitutes either)
- Corn
- Peanuts

Blood testing is available to determine whether or not any of these foods (and many more) are causing you problems. Look for naturopathic or other integrative doctors' test recommendations because these tests are specialized. Your conventional doctor does not use these food allergy panels. The food allergy tests that most conventional MDs perform simply test for IgE reactions, which are the immediate hypersensitivity reactions that you would most likely already know about. The delayed hypersensitivity reactions are the ones we are interested in here and comprise most of the offending results.

One way to test for food allergies or food intolerances without going through a blood test is to do an elimination diet for three weeks, where all the above foods are eliminated in their entirety, and *Whole 30* then add back a food one at a time, leaving 48 hours for delayed reactions to be noticed. IF there is no reaction to the added back food, keep that food in the diet and add the next food. If you notice symptoms such as stomach ache, bloating, gas, indigestion, itchiness of throat, skin eruptions, hives, headache, brain fog, joint pain, fatigue, and heartrate differences, then that food is a problem for you and you would keep that food out of your diet.

As a bonus, people undergoing an elimination diet or removing foods shown to be reactive via a blood test, usually lose weight. My patients call this, and the increased energy "wonderful side effects"!

Food allergies are so important to your overall health, as well as to the health of your skin, that I have included an elimination diet in the **IAMFINE® Facial Rejuvenation Protocol** at the end of the book. Everyone should consider an elimination diet at least once in their life to see what their food allergies or intolerances are. To miss this is to allow hidden inflammation to go on indefinitely in your body. Food allergies are an assault on your immune system. If your body's immune system is unknowingly fighting, let's say corn, on a daily basis, then you are using up valuable immune resources on this food that could be used for other physiological processes such as healing, detoxification, fighting real immune invaders. Food allergies lead to immune dysfunction, which can lead to **autoimmune disease, chronic fatigue, fibromyalgia**, and other chronic diseases.

Food allergies are symptoms of underlying dysfunction in the gut, and once the offending foods are removed, your doctor can prescribe a gut healing protocol. Once you have healed your gut, you may find that those problematic foods don't bother you anymore. A healthy gut should not react to foods.

I was a highly allergic "universal reactor" and asthmatic for my childhood and up to adulthood. I nearly died several times from severe asthma and spent a lot of time in the Emergency Rooms of hospitals. Though I didn't realize it at the time, I was also a terrible detoxifier (validated through genomic testing as an adult), which meant, along with other things, I suffered ALL the side effects of the pharmaceutical drugs I was given to manage my condition.

The discovery by an integrative doctor of my food allergies in my twenties is what **TRANSFORMED** my life by completely exposing what was making me chronically ill. I had never even heard of food allergies and wasn't sure what to make of this doctor, even though I was actively seeking out "alternative medicine," because I felt so miserable under conventional treatment.

I will never forget the day I received the results of my food allergy test. Completely depressed, I made dinner for my husband and dramatically set my own place with a lone rice cracker centered squarely on an otherwise empty plate. I tearfully announced that I could no longer eat any "real" food because of my lengthy list of allergic foods.

Unimpressed by the drama and tears, my level-headed, logical, Naval-officer husband commented that "I had nothing to lose by trying it," and that I could choose from plenty of "real" foods like nearly any vegetable, legumes, and fruit.

I eliminated my allergic foods (which were all the good tasting foods like wheat, eggs, and dairy) and was forced to eat a lot of vegetables, fruits, non-gluten grains, and fish. I was astonished to discover that my health improved, I was able to get off all of my prescription drugs, and my energy skyrocketed. And the best news of all is that my asthma vanished!

This transformative process also propelled me to begin my own journey towards natural health, culminating in going back to naturopathic medical school so that I could similarly help others transform their own lives and recover from chronic disease. Who wants a whole life **DO OVER? Natural medicine is powerful beyond belief and can reverse LIFE-LONG chronic health conditions.** Naturopathic medicine seeks to find the root cause of disease and not merely cover it up with drugs or cut out the offending parts.

Keep Inflammation Down

Keeping the inflammatory transcription factor NFkB low is an excellent way to slow down aging. This can be accomplished through some very specific foods.

Anti-inflammatory foods:

- Fruits and vegetables
- Omega-3 fatty acids
- Olive oil
- Nuts
- Seeds
- Legumes
- Herbs and spices

Foods that fan the flames of inflammation:

- Sugar, sweets
- Processed foods, refined grains, white flour
- Omega-6 fatty acids (soybean, sunflower, other vegetable oils)
- Meats that are feedlot raised and processed
- Trans fats (found in margarine, non-dairy creamers, bakery goods)
- Alcohol —> What? Ouch!

When it comes to the Standard American Diet (the SAD diet), sugar features predominantly. On average, every American consumes about 22 teaspoons of sugar per day. While that may not sound like too much, consider that one can of soda contains just under 10 teaspoons of sugar, 8 ounces of orange juice contains 6 teaspoons, 2 pop tarts boast 8½ teaspoons, and we haven't even gotten to all the processed foods that have sugar (or its evil twin, high fructose corn syrup) added, such as ketchup and barbeque sauce. Even "healthful" items, such as protein bars and granola bars, contain several teaspoons of sugar.

Sugar feeds into the glycation process that we mentioned previously as one route to wrinkle formation. But sugar also feeds directly into the inflammation pathway, which is a one-way street to Wrinkleville. So, by practicing extreme moderation in the sugar department, you are well on your way to having a more youthful-looking complexion.

Processed foods, such as anything made with refined grains, form the bulk of the SAD diet. They are devoid of fiber and vitamin B compared to unpolished and unrefined grains that still have the bran, germ, and the aleurone layer intact. This makes refined grains almost as bad as refined sugars, which are practically empty calories. Refined grains and products made out of them are almost everywhere. The common ones are white rice, white flour, white bread, noodles, pasta, biscuits, and pastries. To make things worse, many products with refined grains undergo further processing to enhance their taste and look, and are often loaded with excess sugar, salt, artificial flavors, and/or partially hydrogenated oil in the process.

A prime example is boxed cereals which contain refined grains that are then bleached, fortified with synthetic vitamins, have substantial amounts of sugar and flavorings added, and are then extruded into fun shapes. This is what most people have for breakfast, and a bagel or toast is not much better. These refined grains rapidly break down into sugar in our bodies, raise our insulin levels, and lead to an energy crash later in the morning. As a nation, we basically are eating dessert for breakfast.

As mentioned previously, Japanese women are notorious for aging gracefully; part of this may be due to their diet. The traditional breakfast in Japan is fish, vegetables, rice, and green tea. It is not a

Super Grandiose Vanilla Sugar Latte with an extra Sugar Shot and a bagel. Consider the relative glycation and inflammation effects from each breakfast, over the course of a lifetime, and it would seem to make sense whose face would wrinkle first.

As far as the omega-3 versus omega-6 fatty-acid content of our diet, it is really the ratio that is important. We need both—that is why they are called essential fatty acids. But the omega-6 fatty acids are so ubiquitous in our diets today that the much higher ratio of omega-6 compared to omega-3 fatty acids now seen, promotes inflammation.

Over the last one hundred years, consumption of omega-6 fatty acids from vegetables oils has risen dramatically, as we did not have the technology to process these oils until then.

So again, including plenty of omega-3 fatty acids in your diet from fatty, low-toxin fish, krill oil, walnuts, chia and flax seeds is a positive for your skin health. Minimizing omega-6 oils, such as the cheap vegetable oils and trans-fats pervasive in processed foods, will also tip your fatty acid profile into the anti-inflammatory category.

Commercially produced meats (which we find in most supermarkets and restaurants) are fed with grains like soy beans and corn—a diet that's high in inflammatory omega-6 fatty acids but low in anti-inflammatory omega-3 fats. In animals, as in humans, the kinds of fats ingested in the diet are then found in the meat because it is true, you are what you eat. So, eating factory farmed meats means you are eating meat that is high in omega-6 fatty acids, the type that promotes inflammation.

Due to their cramped, high-density living environment, these animals also gain excess fat and end up with high levels of saturated fats. Worse, to make the feedlot animals grow faster and prevent them from getting sick, they are also injected with hormones and fed with antibiotics. Processed meat includes animal product that has been smoked, cured, salted, or chemically preserved. Common red meats are beef, lamb, and pork, while processed meats include salami, lunch meat, sausage, and pepperoni.

If you are a meat eater, it is important to eat meat that is of a higher quality. The meat of organic, free-range animals that feed on their natural diet and eat grasses instead of grains and hormones, contain more omega-3 fats. Having more opportunity to roam freely, they are also leaner and contain less saturated fat. When you do eat red meat, remember to choose lean cuts and, preferably, that of grass-fed animals.

In one study in the *Journal of the American College of Nutrition*, it was found that a higher intake of vegetables, legumes, fish, and olive oil appeared to be protective against skin aging. On the other hand, a high intake of meat, dairy, butter, margarine, and sugar promoted skin aging. The vegetables, legumes, fish, and olive oil are pretty much the Mediterranean diet in a nutshell.

Cooking Methods and AGEing

Let's circle back to glycation, the sugar-induced clumping of collagen fibers in your skin. There are two ways to accumulate Advance Glycated Endproducts or AGEs in your body: the first is through sugar intake and the subsequent sugar-induced chemical reaction in our tissues, and the second is through eating preformed

AGEs in our diet. One of the best ways to combat glycation in your skin and body is by paying attention to what you eat and how you cook it. The inhibition of AGE formation through diet and cooking methods is critical to preventing this process from occurring in the first place, as it is largely irreversible. If you can manage your skin AGE production, you will manage your skin's aging. And remember, AGE production in our bodies kicks into high gear once we hit age 35, although it is first observed in skin collagen at age 20.

Low oral consumption of dietary AGEs prevents inflammation and oxidative stress. AGE production also ramps up in the presence of high oxidative stress. Higher AGE intake through the diet is consistently associated with higher blood markers of inflammation. As we know, avoiding inflammation and oxidative stress are crucial to maintaining our youthful skin.

Cooking methods play a strong role in AGE products. Grilling, roasting, searing, and frying accelerate new AGE formation. This "Maillard reaction" occurs during high temperature cooking, causing bonding between glucose molecules and amino acids, which is responsible for the browning of food and the grill marks on grilled meats. Eating foods raw, lightly steamed, or poached, have the lowest AGE production.

Grains, vegetables, legumes, breads, fruits, and milk were among the foods with the lowest amount of dietary AGEs. Fats and meats had the highest amounts of AGEs. Fried foods and highly processed foods accumulate the most AGEs. And, of course, reducing sugar in the diet vastly reduces the formation of AGEs.

Advanced Glycation Endproducts in Some Foods

kU per serving

- Salmon Raw — 475
- Salmon Broiled with Olive Oil — 3,901
- Salmon Poached — 2,063
- Chicken Fried in olive oil — 6,651
- Chicken, breaded and fried — 8,965
- Chicken breast, skinless broiled — 5,245
- Chicken breast poached — 968
- Beef steak, pan-fried, olive oil — 9,052
- Egg fried (one) — 1,237
- Egg Poached (one) — 27
- Bacon, fried 5 min, no extra oil — 11,905
- Avocado — 473
- Celery, raw — 43
- Cucumber, raw — 31
- Green beans, canned — 18
- French Fries (McDonalds) — 1,522
- White potato, boiled — 17

Adapted from Table 1: The advanced glycation endproduct (AGE) content of 549 foods, based on carboxymethyllysine content from J Am Diet Assoc 2010 Jun; 110(6):911-916

A fried egg has 45 times more AGEs than a poached egg. Fried chicken has nearly 7 times the AGEs than poached chicken. The issue is that foods cooked for extended periods of time at high heats with little moisture, are the foods most likely to contribute to your daily load of AGEs. In fact, those lovely brown grilling marks that you see on your grilled steaks and other foods are evidence that let you know the Maillard process, or browning, has occurred. The foods that intrinsically carry more water, like fruits and vegetables, and meats cooked in water, contribute fewer dietary AGEs. Also a cooking process such as a slow cooker which cooks at a lower heat in some sort of fluid, greatly reduces AGEs.

Curiously, however, when omnivores were compared to vegetarians, higher levels of AGEs were found in the vegetarians, despite the fact that animal foods contain higher amounts of AGEs, as you can clearly see in the examples above. According to one study, this was believed to be due to a deficiency in plant foods of the AGE-inhibiting amino acids taurine and carnosine easily found in animal products. According to another study, the vegetarians consumed less protein, but more carbohydrates, and more fructose. Fructose, or fruit sugar found naturally in fruit, honey, and many vegetables (in lower amounts), is a component of table sugar, and is an AGE monster. Fructose is both pro-inflammatory and a strong AGE inducer, which means, if you want to preserve your skin, you will want to avoid excess fructose.

Having said that, most fructose in the diet comes not from actual fruit, but from various processed foods and drinks that are made with high fructose corn syrup (HFCS), or plain sugar. If you look at the ingredient labels on most fruit juices and other processed foods in the supermarket you will quickly learn how prevalent it is in our diet.

To give you an idea of where in our diets fructose is found, I have provided this chart:

Age group	% of fructose from beverages	% of fructose from grains	% of fructose from fruit/juice	% of fructose from sugars/sweets	% of fructose from vegetables	% of fructose from dairy
2-5	27.9	20.1	29.9	9.9	3.6	5.8
6-11	31.3	22.5	19.7	10.4	3.8	9.2
12-18	45.2	20.0	13.0	9.1	3.7	5.6
19-30	43.9	17.8	12.6	8.2	6.2	4.6
31-50	31	21.9	16.3	11.8	7.1	5.5
51-70	18.3	23.1	25.9	11.8	9.3	5.5
>70	8.2	25.3	31.6	13.1	9.1	5.1

Adapted from Medscape J Med 2008; 10(7):160

The article from which the fructose values above are taken states:

"Much attention has focused on sugar-sweetened beverages as a possible source of excess calories. We found that these beverages provide nearly half of the fructose consumed by adolescents (12–18 years) and 30% of fructose for all age groups. Grains (including breads, cereal, cakes, pies, and snacks) were the second-largest source. Breads and cereals alone contributed 12% in children (2–18 years) and 11% in adults. In the very young (2–5 years) and older adults (> 51 years), the category "fruits and 100% fruit juice" was the single largest source of fructose. Notably, for our cohort, *if all sources of fructose were eliminated other than whole fruit and vegetables, children and adults would eliminate 82% and 75% of fructose, respectively.* Our analysis confirms that fructose is prevalent in the American diet and that processed foods in all categories are substantial contributors."

For vegetarians and vegans, an additional step in your skin nutrition protocol might include the amino acids taurine and carnosine in supplement form. See the chapter on Supplements for Beauty to learn about other supplements that can help glycation.

Additionally, vegetarians were found to consume more carbohydrates than those with carnivorous eating habits, and they were found to have a lowered collagen synthesis, by 10%.

Solutions to AGEing

While reversing already formed AGEs in the body continues to elude scientists, studies have elucidated methods of inhibiting their formation, which are not that hard to incorporate into our daily routines.

One way to reduce AGEs in your body is to reduce your consumption of preformed AGEs in your foods. Indeed, this has been borne out in several studies. In one recent study of men, a 12-week diet in which they were simply instructed to follow a routine in which they maintained their usual caloric and nutrient intake, but reduced AGE content by changing cooking methods to lower temperature and higher water content, as in stewing and poaching, was used as an intervention. This group of men was able to lower their blood markers of AGEs by 50% in 12 weeks.

Since we know that AGE formation is intensified in high-oxidative stress environments, maintaining an antioxidant-rich diet is encouraged. Antioxidants are best consumed from vegetables, fruits, and spices.

Controlling blood sugar has also been found to be helpful in controlling production of AGEs.

Certain spices have been found to exhibit very high anti-glycation properties. Ginger appears near the top of this list reducing AGE formation a whopping 93% under experimental conditions. In the same study, cinnamon, a spice favored by people wishing to regulate their blood sugar, came in at a very close second at 88%. Green tea and cumin were also heavy hitters at 86% each.

Conclusion

In terms of skin beauty, you really are what you eat. Your skin is a reflection of the health and beauty that is present on the inside. Another way to look at it is that your food choices actually *create* your beauty. In order to achieve radiant, glowing, smooth, and youthful-looking skin, it is best to choose whole, organic, plant foods that provide antioxidants that fight free radicals and repair your skin, and enable your body to produce its own antioxidants and strengthen its defenses against aging. Furthermore, avoiding processed foods, sugars, and other foods that enhance inflammation, and achieving a balance of healthy fats in your diet, will reduce inflammation and the damage done to your skin. With the right dietary choices, your skin will truly shine and represent your best self to the outside world!

The most beneficial foods for your skin, which were explained in more detail earlier in the chapter, are listed below.

Top 7 Foods for Skin Rejuvenation:
- Green tea
- Broccoli, kale
- Olive oil
- Berries
- Wild salmon or alternate source of omega-3 fatty acids
- Walnuts
- Avocado

Another easy way to give your skin a nutritional jolt is by juicing. Juicing positively saturates your body with easily absorbed nutrients. Here is my favorite juice recipe that enhances skin health and beauty.

Dr. Fine's Skin Beauty Juice Recipe

All items are best organic; otherwise you are simply concentrating pesticides into a glass, and then drinking them.

- 1 carrot (optional for those with sugar issues)
- 4 stalks of celery
- 1 large handful parsley
- 1 large handful spinach
- ¼ beet
- 1-2 inches of ginger (can work your way up)
- 1-2 cloves of garlic (occasionally, not every day)
- 1/3 cucumber
- ½ lemon

Applying the information

The Minimalist

- Switch out your coffee for skin enhancing **green tea**. Brew a cup or more at home and drink there or put into an insulated stainless steel cup to bring to work
- Add a serving of organic fresh or frozen **berries** to your breakfast, or throw into a smoothie. If you are using frozen berries, take a serving out of the bag and put into a bowl on

your countertop or in your refrigerator before you go to bed, so it will be defrosted by morning.

- Add half of an **avocado** to your diet each day.

The Middle Way: Accompanying the above,

- Add 2 or more servings of cruciferous vegetables per day
- Add the Dr. Fine Beauty Juice to your daily diet
- Switch out fried foods for poaching in water or other liquid

The Beauty Buff: In Addition to All of the above,

- Go on the **Elimination Diet: eliminate all on this list for 21 days**
    - o Wheat/gluten
    - o Dairy
    - o Eggs
    - o Soy
    - o Sugar (don't use sugar substitutes either)
    - o Peanuts
    - o Corn

These are some clear examples of nutrigenomics at work. In the rest of the book we will take a look at how our environment affects our skin health and beauty. Are there choices that we can make every day that enhance our skin beauty? You bet there are. Keep reading to find out what you can do starting now, at home, to protect your skin against premature aging, wrinkles, rashes, eruptions, loss of radiance and elasticity, and sagging.

CHAPTER FOUR

Supplements for Beauty

"The Beauty-From-Within Trend is here to stay and nutricosmetics will soon become a buzzword in the world of beauty"—**Dr. Fine**

YOUR SKIN IS BOTH NOURISHED AND HYDRATED from within, and also is affected by its environment without. While a healthy, clean diet rich in nutrient density is a must for healthy skin, certain supplements can contribute to an even better glow. Part of the reason supplements are so useful for skin is that our current diets are inferior in quality to the whole foods diet that our ancestors ate, and part of it is from the fact that our soils are so deficient in minerals that our crops, even the organic ones, do not contain nearly as many nutrients as they did even 50 years ago.

A landmark study was published in the *Journal of the American College of Nutrition* in 2004 regarding nutritional value of fruits and vegetables. They studied U.S. Department of Agriculture nutritional data from both 1950 and 1999 for 43 different vegetables and fruits and found "reliable declines" in the amount of protein, calcium, phosphorus, iron, riboflavin, and vitamin C over the last half century.

Vitamin C, for example, is absolutely critical for making collagen in the skin. We are always turning over our skin and other tissues, and remaking collagen in our skin. Our bodies cannot make collagen without vitamin C. Since we do not make vitamin C in our bodies, we must always have a ready supply.

William Albrecht, a soil scientist and visionary from the early part of the twentieth century, looked into soil quality decades ago. He believed that people and animals provide a "biochemical photograph" of the soils in which their foods have grown. With effective and affordable commercial fertilizers that became available after World War II, the common wisdom felt that attention to soil health and productivity was no longer necessary. A half-century later America is facing an epidemic of diet-related illnesses including obesity, diabetes, heart disease, hypertension, and various cancers, even though efficiencies in crop production were achieved. Recent scientific studies have linked a decrease in nutritional density in food to declining health in the soils in which they are grown, resulting in foods that are calorie-rich, but nutrient-poor. As it turns out, Albrecht was a visionary in the sustainable movement long before sustainability became a buzz word.

The declining nutrient portfolio in foods grown with modern agriculture, meaning a loss of vitamins, minerals, good fats, and phytonutrients, is why I believe supplementation is beneficial for most people. Of course, quality is paramount with any substance that you take into the body, and not all supplements are created equal. I recommend professional lines of supplements that are carried by your naturopathic or integrative physician, along with professional guidance on what you should be taking. Don't rely on Dr. Google for your healthcare or nutritional needs. See a doctor who can have lab testing done that will reveal deficiencies or excesses and properly assess your health concerns.

Once, while I was an intern, I saw a patient who had what could only be described as "chicken skin." Her skin, all over her body, had a distinctly yellowish cast to it and was puckery and rubbery. I was also surprised that she appeared several *decades* older than her stated age. I had never seen anything like it. As part of my initial intake, I always ask about diet. So the diet part of the interview went something like this:

Dr. Fine: How many servings of fruits and vegetables do you eat in a day?

Patient: None.

Dr. Fine: None, really? Ever?

Patient: Nope. I don't like them. Never have.

Dr. Fine: Hmmmm...well, how many glasses of water do you drink in a day?

Patient: None.

Dr. Fine: I see. What do you normally drink, then?

Patient: Diet coke...all day.

Dr. Fine: Could you tell me what you would eat for breakfast on a normal day?

Patient: Diet coke and potato chips.

This patient was also so severely constipated that she required manual evacuation on a regular basis and simply could not "go" on her own. In this patient, several themes emerge that potentially contributed to her bad skin condition. Constipation, which changes the gut flora, or microbiota, which has an effect on the skin; lack of water/hydration; complete lack of fresh, whole fruits and vegetables, which means no nutrition to get into her skin cells; and finally, a diet consisting of 100% processed food containing bad fats, additives, preservatives, MSG, and no nutritional value whatsoever. By far, this was the starkest example of "you are what you eat" that I have ever seen, likely made worse by the impact of this diet on her particular genetic profile, resulting in this rare skin condition. Remember, genes load the gun, but environment pulls the trigger.

Antioxidants for Skin

If you look at the skin aging graphic from Chapter One again, you can see that one of the precipitating events for skin aging is the formation of reactive oxygen species, or free radicals, which occurs both in intrinsic and extrinsic aging. So to successfully outsmart the aging process, clearly, antioxidants would be of value since they mop up free radicals before they can inflict their damage.

Antioxidant superstars, such as vitamins A, C, and E, have been studied for their skin-health benefits for many decades.

Vitamin A has been widely studied and considered a great ally, showing both anti-acne effects and anti-aging effects. It has also been shown to be helpful for eliminating dry, scaly, and flaky skin. Vitamin A and its derivatives, retinoids and carotenoids, can be found in both animal and plant foods. But if you have digestive issues, like Celiac or Crohn's disease, irritable bowel syndrome (IBS), or pancreatic diseases and deficiencies of certain enzymes, you may not be absorbing this important fat-soluble vitamin. This is an important point, because when digestive health is intact, it is easy to get all the vitamin A you need from your diet, and supplementing it could be detrimental.

The retinoids are mostly found in animal sources, while the carotenoids, which are converted to vitamin A, are found mostly in plant products. Beta-carotene is a common carotenoid found in orange-colored plant foods like carrots and sweet potatoes. As it turns out, skin is one of the most active locations for retinoid receptors. Previous studies have discovered roles for retinoids in the skin as useful for enhancing repair of UV-damaged skin, their ability to increase the proliferation of new skin cells, their ability to inhibit the MMPs, matrix-degrading enzymes, which results in preservation of tissue collagen and elastin in the skin making it appear healthy and young.

How many of you have noticed red bumpy skin on the backs of your arms or the arms of your children? This is one sign of a possible vitamin A deficiency. As vitamin A is easily found in the diet, malabsorption syndromes should be evaluated.

Supplementation with vitamin A alone is not recommended, unless under the supervision of your physician. Too much vitamin A has been shown to be detrimental to your health, even causing birth defects in pregnant mothers. It is much better to get your vitamin A from the carotenoid family found in dark leafy greens, carrots, cantaloupe, and sweet potatoes. The body then converts these beta-carotenes into vitamin A. There has never been a documented problem in someone getting too much vitamin A from eating too many fruits and vegetables

Vitamin C is absolutely critical for making collagen in the skin. We are always turning over our skin and other tissues, and remaking collagen in our skin. Our bodies cannot make collagen without vitamin C. Since we do not make vitamin C in our bodies, we must always have a ready supply. Collagen is what fills out our wrinkles.

Recall from our previous discussion of UV irradiation from the sun how damaging it is for our skin. Excessive exposure to UV irradiation causes photoaging and can result in the development of skin cancer. UV irradiation induces reactive oxygen species (free radicals or ROS), suppresses the expression of a factor that promotes collagen formation, and induces the expression of the MMPs, the enzymes that break down collagen and elastin in the skin. So, if you are suppressing the formation of collagen and increasing its breakdown, the result will be wrinkles, coarse texture, and laxity—not a pretty picture. Vitamin C has been shown to significantly suppress the UV light-triggered production of free radicals, protecting cells from oxidative stress leading to skin aging. In addition, it increases collagen synthesis, improves skin hydration levels, and has wound healing properties.

Definitely include vitamin C in your skin-care routine as it will be one of the powerhouses in maintaining your youthful skin.

Vitamin E is a fat-soluble antioxidant. Even one single dose of UV irradiation can deplete the amount of vitamin E in the skin, making it a very sensitive marker of oxidative stress in the human skin. Vitamin E has a number of properties, such as it reduces lipid peroxidation, photoaging, immunosuppression, and skin cancer caused by the sun. Lipid peroxidation is the term given to oxidizing fat, and our skin does contain fat. Lipid peroxidation is fat oxidation which degrades cells and is a part of skin aging.

In addition to the antioxidant properties listed above, vitamin E attenuates skin inflammation, also a prime contributor to skin aging. This is because tocotrienols also downregulate the Master Switch for pro-inflammatory genes, NF-kB, thereby short-circuiting the wrinkle cascade.

Natural vitamin E really refers to an entire family of vitamin E products: four tocopherols and four tocotrienols. Alpha-tocopherol is the form most frequently found in vitamin supplements and has the most studies behind it. But recently, much attention and focus has centered around the four tocotrienols for their multifaceted benefits that extend beyond their function as antioxidants. Specifically for the skin, tocotrienols have been found to be useful in preventing oxidative stress-induced skin aging by modulating the changes in total collagen synthesis and expression of *COL I*, *COL III* and *COL IV* genes; the genes that make collagen. In cell culture studies, total collagen and the collagen genes were all upregulated and collagen breakdown enzymes (the MMPs) were inhibited, resulting in more collagen in the skin.

In addition, tocotrienols have been found to lengthen telomeres, the protective caps on the ends of DNA strands that shorten with age. Every time your cell replicates, these telomeres get a little bit shorter, until the cells are no longer able to divide and so they die. Longer telomeres mean younger cells. This means tocotrienols have the ability to fight against oxidative stress-induced telomere shortening which results in aging. Adding tocotrienols to your beauty supplement plan can protect your skin and telomeres.

Tocotrienols provide potent anti-aging and rejuvenating benefits to your skin by protecting your skin against free-radical damage, while simultaneously boosting the production of collagen to plump up your wrinkles, and actually extending the length of telomeres while preventing damage to DNA. All told, tocotrienols are veritable candidates for the Fountain of Youth.

These antioxidants work together synergistically and studies bear this out. Taken alone, they do not appear to positively influence skin quality; but taken together they have been found to offer UV protection and support better skin health.

Vitamin D is very important for skin health and wound healing as well. One of its primary roles is to stimulate the skin's innate antimicrobial defense system. I bet you didn't know that your skin contains its own antimicrobial arsenal. But it makes sense in that, many threats to the human body initiate at the level of skin through things we touch, for example.

Vitamin D is a vitamin that we can make in our own bodies. The skin contains vitamin D receptors that are triggered by UV radiation to start the vitamin D production process. The process of converting the sun's rays to vitamin D in the body begins on the skin, travels through the blood to our liver, and then to our kidneys. Vitamin D has many functions on our bodies, many of them having to do with the absorption of calcium in our intestines and bone health, and others with our immune system.

As vitamin D is not very abundant in foods, with the exception of some fish (cod liver oil is the highest source of vitamin D from food) and fortified foods, exposing the skin to the sun for a limited time each day, or taking a good vitamin D supplement is highly recommended.

I have been testing vitamin D levels in my patients for over ten years and am always shocked at how low my Arizona and California patients are in vitamin D, even though they live in sun-drenched areas and make a point of getting some sunshine every day.

As vitamin D is a fat-soluble vitamin and can be stored in the body, it is imperative to test your blood for vitamin-D levels before considering supplementing. More and more doctors are testing for vitamin D and recommending supplementation as the benefits of vitamin D continue to be discovered.

Zinc also has an important role to play in maintaining skin health. Its main function is to protect the skin against photodamage by the sun by absorbing UV irradiation. Zinc is also necessary for proper wound healing. As well, zinc has been found to be a valuable ally in addressing acne.

Copper is an essential trace mineral that also acts like an antioxidant. Copper is necessary to stimulate the maturity of collagen, making it a critical ingredient in preserving the elasticity and thickness of skin.

Selenium, another trace mineral, also protects the skin from UV radiation by stimulating selenium-dependent antioxidant enzymes. These enzymes turn on the body's ability to make its own antioxidants—something far more clever than having to rely on continuous intake of other antioxidants. Selenium deficiency has also been noted in some skin diseases such as psoriasis and is associated with an increased risk of skin cancer.

Key Vitamins and Micronutrients in Skin Health

Vitamin A

- Modulates hyper-proliferation of skin cells
- Prevents UV radiation-mediated skin damage
- Prevents and treats psoriasis, ichthyosis, acne, and cancer

Vitamin C

- Protects cells from oxidative stress triggered by UV radiation
- Wound healing, necessary for collagen formation
- Increases epidermal moisture levels increasing skin hydration

Vitamin D

- Improves innate immunity
- Decreases inflammation
- Wound healing
- Anticancer

Vitamin E

- Decreases lipid peroxidation
- Modulates photoaging
- Anti-inflammatory

Zinc

- Protects from photodamage
- Exhibits antimicrobial activity

Copper

- Antioxidant
- Stimulates maturation of collagen
- Modulates melanin synthesis

Selenium

- Protects skin from UV radiation-induced oxidative stress

Moisturizing from Within

Did you know that your skin is actually hydrated from within? You can put a moisturizer on your skin and it will feel hydrated, but that is because the moisturizer is effectively reducing the amount of moisture evaporating from the skins surface. This is called trans-epidermal water loss (TEWL). The higher your TEWL is, the drier your skin will be. The real moisturizing effects come from within the body. This is why drinking water is so good for the skin, and why flying, which is very deydrating, makes the skin look bad.

For this reason, drinking enough water and staying properly hydrated is a mainstay of having great skin. You must replenish the amount of moisture evaporating from your skin on a constant basis. Avoid dehydrating beverages, such as caffeinated beverages and alcohol, or drink two cups of water for every cup of coffee or alcohol to replenish what you lost. A good rule of thumb for hydration is to drink half your body weight in ounces of water every day; do not count caffeinated beverages or alcohol in that amount.

If you are going to be drinking alcohol, intersperse a glass of water in between every drink in order to maintain hydration, and include another glass of water before going to bed. Part of the ill effects of a hangover is simply the effects of dehydration.

Fats

The quality and quantity of fats in your diet also have a large influence on the quality of your skin hydration and health. Chronic inflammation, which is caused by a number of factors, such as poor diets high in the wrong kind of fats and deficient in the right kind of fats, and sugar, drives aging and wrinkle formation. This is why taking certain oils and fats are good for the skin, while certain other fats are bad.

Omega-3 fatty acids are found in fish oil, walnuts, flaxseeds, and chia seeds. They are anti-inflammatory as well as hydrating to the skin.

People who are on low-fat diets often have very dry skin. There are also some people who consume fats, but do not absorb them very well. Perhaps they have malabsorption or a gastrointestinal disease like inflammatory bowel disease.

But the topic of essential fatty acids for wrinkle modulation requires some explanation; otherwise you will not know WHICH kind of oil to get for its skin-health benefits.

In Chapter One, we discussed how chronic inflammation leads to wrinkles. The primary culprit produced during inflammation that degrades the collagen is called PGE2, one of the prostaglandins, an entire family of inflammatory substances. In studies it has been reliably linked to skin aging.

PGE2 turns on the matrix metalloproteinases (MMPs) that we have talked about, which are damaging and degrading your collagen fibers. Also PGE2 has the ability to inhibit formation of new collagen by our fibroblasts, the skin cells that actually make new collagen, a double tragedy with respect to beautiful skin since it is both damaging the collagen and inhibiting its replenishment.

Ultraviolet rays have been shown to increase the levels of PGE2 formation in the skin. New research shows that, in particular, UVA rays, the ones that penetrate deep into your skin dermis and literally turn ON aging, really cause an increase in inflammatory PGE2.

While the connection between UV rays and skin aging, or photoaging, is known, what is not well known is that the kinds of fat we eat influence skin aging as well. Excess vegetable oils have also been found to turn on PGE2 and lead to inflammation and aging.

There are two kinds of essential fatty acids: omega-3 and omega-6. They are called essential because our bodies cannot make them. Omega-6 essential fatty acids are derived from vegetable oils such as corn, soybean, sunflower, and safflower oil, which are linoleic-acid-rich vegetable oils. They are mostly considered pro-inflammatory because they increase production of PGE2 in the skin. However, they are still essential for human health. Pro-inflammatory means more wrinkles. Since they are both necessary for human health, it is the ratio of omega-6 to omega-3 that is important for human health and the health of our skin, which is more favorable if the balance of omega-6 to omega-3 is not too high. Having more omega-6 fatty acids in our bodies is normal and desirable, and certain omega-6 fatty acids, such as borage and evening primrose oil, can be helpful for certain skin conditions.

Unfortunately, omega-6 essential fatty acids are the primary fat in the diets of North Americans and have now increased to three times more per person today, than in 1960. Soybean oil consumption alone has increased 1000% from 1909 to 1999, according to the *American Journal of Clinical Nutrition* in 2011. That's a lot of pro-inflammatory stimulation of PGE2 for millions of unsuspecting Americans. This huge increase of vegetable oil takes its toll on collagen.

In the United States, oils from corn and soybeans are found in most fast and processed foods, and in the feed given to domesticated animals used for meat and dairy products. When these fats are eaten by the animals, the meat contains the same fats. So if you are eating commercially raised beef, which is raised on a greater ratio of omega 6 oils, you are getting the same higher ratio of omega-6 fats in your diet. The Standard American Diet, high in processed foods, contains a higher ratio of omega-6 fatty acids to omega-3 fatty acids, which means it is pro-inflammatory. This is also the reason why embarking on a whole foods diet (paleo, vegetarian, blood type diet, etc.) tends to make people healthier—the diets all restrict or eliminate processed foods, which are high in the omega-6 fatty acids.

By way of contrast, omega-3 essential fatty acids are anti-inflammatory. Consume these oils and you will turn OFF NF-kappa B, a main transcription factor that turns on inflammation, and reduce the MMPs and AP-1, factors involved in the degradation of collagen. This translates into less wrinkling.

One only has to look in the literature at the Inuit population to gather some interesting facts about omega-3 fats derived from their high seafood diet and their skin health. In the first part of the twentieth century, some medical doctors who lived with the Inuit observed that their skin was free of acne blemishes and youthful looking. But once the Western diet was introduced into their lives, including lots of omega-6 fats, sugar, and processed foods, their rates of acne shot up. Acne is another inflammatory disorder of the skin.

As knowledge and interest in omega-3 fish oils cranked up in the 1970s, researchers found that the Inuit, who still consumed more fatty fish than other populations, consistently reported lower rates of psoriasis and other skin diseases, including skin cancer.

A groundbreaking study published in 1992 showed for the first time that, if you gave fish oil to adults (2.8 grams daily), an SPF factor equivalent to 1.15 was obtained. While this sounds like too little to make a difference, over a lifetime of consistent intake, this would result in a 30 percent reduction of lifetime risk of skin cancer. Now that is significant!

Fish oil may also be useful for preventing UV-induced, non-melanoma skin cancer. A growing body of evidence from experimental and clinical studies supports that the use of dietary omega-3 fatty acids inhibits the UV-induced skin damage that leads to skin cancer. Interestingly, it seems to do this through significantly reducing the levels of PGE2 in UV-radiated human skin.

What about the dreaded problem of sagging skin and loss of firmness? The loss of a sharp jawline and general looseness of skin are also unwelcome signs of aging. Can fish oil do anything for elasticity?

One small study published in the *Journal of Dermatological Research* in 2008 looked at fish oil for skin elasticity. Women who were supplemented with only a little over a gram of fish oil for three months, which is easily obtained, demonstrated improvement in the elasticity of their skin. Elasticity was increased by 10%, which, although small, was a significant improvement over the control group of women. And in the absence of any intervention, elasticity will simply decline with time.

More recently, a clinical study utilizing a combination oral supplement for the evaluation of wrinkle reduction in women found that a supplement drink containing soy isoflavones, lycopene, vitamins C and E, given along with a fish oil pill containing less than one gram of EPA and DHA, had a significant effect on wrinkle reduction, particularly the deeper wrinkles, and also increased the deposition of new collagen fibers in the dermis. I want to highlight the significance of the deeper wrinkles being more amenable to fish oil intervention. When we eat or take a supplement for skin health and beauty, it first passes through the digestive system, is taken up into the bloodstream, and then reaches the dermis first, before passing up to the epidermis. It demonstrates the beauty from the inside-out approach beautifully, because the dermis, which lies underneath the epidermis, is where the deep wrinkles are.

What has happened over the human span of development and evolution is that our ratio of omega-6 to omega-3, which was for much of human evolution about 2-3:1, has now been pushed, just in the last 100 years or so, to about 20-30:1. This ten-fold increase of omega-6 fats has deleterious effects on our body, including on our skin. Chronic inflammation now bears the brunt of fueling much of what ails mankind today: chronic inflammatory diseases such as autoimmune disease, asthma, inflammatory bowel diseases such as Crohn's and Ulcerative Colitis, and skin conditions such as psoriasis.

The dose of fish oil helpful for a skin-beautifying effect is about 1 gram per day of EPA and DHA. The current daily intake of EPA and DHA in the United States is a paltry 130 mg. But please know how to read the fish oil label so that you know how much EPA and DHA you are actually getting in your dose, because the label will list two different amounts for fish oil: one the actual amount of *fish oil* in the serving, and then underneath it, the actual amount of EPA and DHA that you will get, which is always less than the first number.

Of course, consult with your own physician first before adding any supplement. In the case of fish oil, thinner blood is achieved, which may not be good for you if you are on other blood thinners or are taking other medications that may interfere with blood clotting.

Furthermore, not all fish oils are created equal, and it is important to get the right one. Fish oils, as with any fats, are subject to rancidity. Rancid fats of any type are not going to be beneficial. It is best for the fish oil to have some form of antioxidant in it such as vitamin E or astaxanthin. Also, fish oils may come from highly contaminated fish and contain PCBs, heavy metals, dioxins, and other industrial pollutants. Purchase a fish oil whose manufacturer has purified the fish oil from these contaminants and has been third party tested for purity.

Before we leave this discussion of essential fats, I need to point out that omega-6 fatty acids are so prevalent in the diet, that there is rarely any need to supplement them, even though they are also essential fatty acids. However, there is one kind of omega-6 fat that is very good for the skin and does not raise skin-inflammatory PGE2. It is called gamma-linolenic acid, or GLA. GLA is found in borage, evening primrose, and black-currant seed oil; it is not very prevalent in other foods. GLA has actually been shown to turn down the degradation of collagen by PGE2, in direct contrast to its omega-6 fatty cousins.

GLA also helps with hydration of skin by reducing water evaporation through the epidermis, and it only takes about two months to notice this effect. As well, it can diminish dry, itchy skin, a result of deficient internal moisturization from proper fats.

Combining GLA from borage oil and fish or krill oil is a smart way to start providing proper fats for your age-defying skin.

And finally, a word about flax oil, a mainstay in health-food stores all over the world, source of omega-3 essential fatty acids, AND from a vegetarian source. While flax oil DOES contain more omega-3 than omega-6, it is in a form called alpha-linolenic acid or ALA, and requires in the human body an enzyme called delta-six desaturase to convert it into the usable forms: EPA and DHA. And unfortunately, this enzyme does not work very well in adults, particularly those on the Western diet. You will probably do much better with a source of preformed EPA and DHA such as found in fish oil or oily fish. Vegans and vegetarians can source EPA and DHA from microalgae.

Beauty Boost

Fish Oil

- Anti-inflammatory
- Increases elasticity
- Moisturizing
- Inhibits UV-induced damage

Carotenoids

Carotenoids are another antioxidant powerhouse that can help promote youthful skin. Carotenoids mop up free radicals, decrease the inflammation driver, NF-kappa B, induce our own body's production of antioxidants and detoxifying enzymes, Nrf-2 (lycopene only), and decrease MMPs, the enzymes that break down our collagen and produce wrinkles.

Where are these miraculous little nutrients found? They are the yellow-orange pigments found in sweet potatoes, carrots, tomatoes, pumpkin, cantaloupe, and apricots, and are also found in watermelon, dark leafy greens, and broccoli. But some of these nutrients need to be ingested orally in supplement form in order to achieve the dosage required that has been shown to be effective.

Need Supplent?

Dark leafy greens contain a very beneficial antioxidant called lutein, which helps quench free radicals that damage your skin. Lutein is found abundantly in watercress, parsley, kale, broccoli, and spinach. Another carotenoid antioxidant found in the yellow-orange vegetables, such as corn and bell peppers, and goji berries is zeaxanthin. These two carotenoids are known for their benefits to eye health and skin beauty and protection from UV-induced damage.

Technically, zeaxanthin and lutein belong to a class of carotenoids known as xanthophylls. Xanthophylls serve as natural sunscreens in plants, protecting them from the damaging effects of excessive light-derived energy; in humans they may provide the same sun protection benefits.

One Italian study clearly showed an improvement in skin hydration in humans in a fast 21 days from consuming a supplement containing 6 mg lutein and 0.3 mg zeaxanthin daily. This study also explained the mechanism on how that worked. These two antioxidants actually increased the fats in the outer layer of the skin and improved the skin-barrier function and hydration through the decrease in trans-epidermal water loss, an effect that goes well beyond the antioxidant effects for which they are known.

Astaxanthin is a newcomer to the oral, anti-aging, skin-care regime. In fact, it works like an internal beauty pill. Astaxanthin is a strongly antioxidant, xanthophyll carotenoid that is widely found in marine life—shrimp, crab, salmon and, yes, flamingos, who consume the algae from which this is produced. Indeed, it is the pigment which gives these sea creatures their pink color.

Algae named *Haematococcus pluvialis* make astaxanthin only when their water supply dries up and they need to protect themselves from the sun. It is a plant defense molecule and, perhaps not surprisingly, astaxanthin acts like an internal sunscreen when taken by people.

It has potent antioxidant and anti-inflammatory properties, with 10-fold greater antioxidant action than that of other carotenoids and 100-fold greater action than that of α-tocopherol, one of the vitamin E isomers. And vitamin E is considered a skin superstar supplement!

Astaxanthin has been found to protect against UV radiation in skin cells while also inhibiting skin pigmentation. It does this by downregulating the MMPs, the collagen-eating enzymes induced by UV radiation, and by downregulating inflammatory mediators, while also quenching free radicals. Free radicals, MMPs, and inflammation lead to wrinkling, so, inhibiting wrinkling along with preventing age spots makes astaxanthin a multifunctioning, beauty-from-within supplement.

Combining astaxanthin with collagen provided even more skin beauty-boosting effects. In one human clinical study, participants ingested either an oral supplement containing 2 mg astaxanthin and 3 g collagen hydrolysate or a placebo daily for 12 weeks. After 12 weeks, the elasticity and barrier integrity of the astaxanthin/collagen hydrolysate group showed significant improvement compared with the placebo group. In addition, collagen genes were turned on and Matrix Metalloproteinases (MMPs) were turned down.

Collagen supplementation alone has also been found to have anti-aging benefits to the face. It is often used in combination supplements for the skin, as well.

Very recently, two clinical trials were conducted evaluating collagen peptides (prepared in a 10-gram drink) consumed orally by women between the ages of 40 and 65. Skin hydration was significantly improved by week 8 (28% more moisture as compared to placebo), and skin collagen density increased by 4 weeks into the study by 9% as compared to placebo. Furthermore, it was revealed that the collagen peptides induced collagen formation as well as production of extracellular matrix (to better plump up your skin), and turned down the collagen-eating MMPs, which reduced collagen fragmentation in the skin. Moisture content in skin, collagen levels, collagen breakdown—these are all the hallmarks of skin aging that were elegantly shown to be positively affected by the addition of a collagen peptide supplement.

Probiotics

People are often very surprised to hear that there is a strong relationship between gastrointestinal health and their skin. The digestive system is much more than just a food processing plant. About 70% of your immune system is located in your gut. And did you know there are so many neurons that reside in your gut, it is considered a "second brain"? Skin health and its condition are representative of what is going on in the body—and health begins in the gut.

There is a lot going on in your digestive tract that can affect your skin. Let's take a look.

The microbiota, formerly known as microflora or flora, has become a hot research interest lately. There are trillions of bacteria colonizing our gut, outnumbering our human cells. The good ones are very busy producing vitamins, undergoing detoxification and metabolism, stimulating the immune response, and helping to keep the bad bacteria in check. In the early twentieth century, some bacteria in the gut were hypothesized to actually produce some beneficial compounds that could protect against premature aging. This discovery set off the whole probiotic culture, as researchers and doctors started identifying these beneficial, good bacteria strains and producing orally administered forms of them to patients.

More recent research on probiotics has demonstrated that orally administered probiotics have decreased skin inflammation in skin conditions such as eczema and acne. More wide-ranging skin effects have been shown as probiotics have also been found to decrease the inflammation-promoting and collagen-destroying chemicals called cytokines, all over the body. This has implications for skin health, but also for inflammation-related disease throughout the body, including arthritis.

Orally ingested probiotics have also been shown to attenuate the damage to skin by UV rays—a unique finding that contributes to our understanding of skin health as a reflection of internal gastrointestinal physiology.

In 2015, a randomized, double-blind, placebo-controlled study was carried out on 110 women between the ages of 41 and 59. A probiotic was given once a day to the active group and the control group received a placebo for 12 weeks. Daily intake of the probiotic was found to significantly increase skin moisture, reduce wrinkling, and improve skin elasticity as compared to the control group. The skin elasticity alone increased by 22% in 12 weeks. That's a fantastic result from a simple study on probiotics' impact on skin aging.

This study built on a previous study in mice where it was discovered that the same probiotic regulated the expression of a gene related to skin hydration—the very definition of epigenetics—and also suppressed the UV radiation-induced molecular signaling within the skin cells. This is the very essence of an anti-aging, nutricosmetic agent and a very exciting finding for the future of skin care.

Constipation is very prevalent in our society and, since the skin is an organ of elimination, toxins that are not eliminated in the stool simply get reabsorbed into your blood stream and attempt to exit through the skin. If this becomes a chronic condition, which so often it does, eruptions, rashes, and poor quality skin can result.

Constipation, when it becomes chronic, reduces beneficial gut bacteria (with lower levels of *Lactobacilli* and *Bifidobacteria*), sharply increases gut permeability, and provokes something truly terrible for the skin: the manufacture of collagen-destroying inflammatory molecules, thus resulting in premature aging of the skin and poor quality skin. Probiotics can help with constipation.

Another concept that will help explain the gut-skin connection is something called intestinal permeability. The intestinal wall cellular junctions are supposed to be so tight, that nothing on the inside of the intestines is supposed to get to the outside via the blood stream. However, when intestinal permeability is present, toxins from the bowel, which include bacteria, leak out and systemically present to the rest of the body, causing extra-intestinal (outside the intestine) symptoms such as migraine headaches, autoimmune disease, arthritis, skin rashes, skin blemishes, and poor quality skin.

Chronic constipation, disordered gut flora, sugar and alcohol consumption, food allergies, antibiotic use, and stress all lead to gut permeability, often called leaky gut, and also small intestinal bacterial overgrowth (SIBO). Symptoms of SIBO can include bloating and abdominal pain, constipation or diarrhea, gas, and fatigue. Both lead to accelerated aging of the skin via increased inflammatory molecules that reach the skin.

One example of an inflammatory skin condition linked to bacteria in the gut is acne rosacea, a facial acne syndrome that includes redness and small red lines over the cheeks and nose of the face, along with pimples. It is often treated with a triple antibiotic therapy aimed at eradicating bacteria. One theory is that *Helicobacter pylori* is the culprit. Another links rosacea to small intestinal bacterial overgrowth (SIBO). SIBO has been found to be ten times as prevalent in people with acne rosacea compared to healthy controls. Correction of SIBO has led to marked improvement in acne rosacea.

While the American Academy of Dermatologists (AAD), in 2013, proposed the use of probiotics in treating rosacea and small trials have shown promising results using probiotics, in my own practice, I have not observed the administration of probiotics as a standalone therapy to be sufficient for the eradication of acne rosacea; although it helps. The area of gut microbiota continues to accrue expanded research efforts that highlight the complexity of our intestinal bacterial milieu, and how it relates to the rest of our body. It is fascinating work and sure to yield new revelations and applications in the future.

One such study, in three separate, randomized, double-blind, placebo-controlled interventions, has demonstrated that, in only 8 weeks, daily administration of a particular probiotic strain, *Bifidobacteria infantis* (*B. infantis*) 35624, reduced the 3 inflammatory markers studied in 70% of patients presenting with psoriasis, ulcerative colitis, and chronic fatigue syndrome. 70%! The fact that our microbiota modulates our immune system and systemically reduces inflammation outside of our guts is still a relatively new concept, but one that can be used to support robust health in our skin. Multiple studies have demonstrated the reduction in inflammatory cytokines in skin conditions such as eczema and acne. Remember, these inflammatory cytokines are also able to wreak havoc on our collagen, literally breaking them down.

Do you have sensitive skin? Sensitive skin is found in skin conditions like atopic dermatitis, contact dermatitis, psoriasis, acne rosacea, and urticaria (hives). It describes skin which is overly sensitive to chemicals (think topically applied products such as soaps and skin care products), temperature, and wind, and implies a problem in the barrier function of the skin. Another probiotic strain was tested in sensitive skin volunteers in a double-blind study, and the results indicated that, in the probiotic group, skin sensitivity decreased, along with trans-epidermal water loss, meaning that the skin was more moisturized, both indicative of improved skin-barrier function, which is so critical to our skin health.

Orally ingested probiotics have also been shown to attenuate the damage to skin by UV rays—a unique finding that further contributes to our understanding of skin health as a reflection of internal gastrointestinal physiology.

Probiotic strains are not all created equally. It is very important to take the highest-quality probiotic. The probiotics available on the shelves of your local health-food store may not contain the stated label amounts of the bacteria listed on the label—there may not even be any viable bacteria species in the entire bottle. Probiotics are alive and must be handled and shipped very carefully to preserve the viability of the bacterial strains. There is no way for the consumer to know if they are buying a good product. I highly recommend professional lines of supplements, including probiotics, which can be obtained from your naturopathic physician or other integrative health specialist.

> # Beauty Boost
>
> Probiotics
>
> - Improve constipation
> - Improve imbalances of good and bad bacteria in gut
> - Decrease inflammation, protect collagen
> - Improve skin-barrier function
> - Assist in skin conditions such as acne, psoriasis, acne rosacea

Methylsulfonylmethane (MSM) is a sulfur-containing molecule that has known beneficial effects for pain relief and inflammation and, wrinkles. Sulfur is an essential part of all connective tissue, including collagen. Sulfur is found in keratin, which means it is found in our skin, hair, and nails. A constant supply of sulfur is necessary to continuously build and rebuild our collagen and keratin in our bodies to keep our hair, nails, and skin strong, radiant, and beautiful. In fact, adding MSM to your protocol will make your nails grow faster and stronger, and your hair and skin more lustrous. Sulfur is also involved in the detoxification pathways of our cells—it helps take out the garbage—and functions as a strong anti-inflammatory, making it good for pain reduction. Sulfur makes your skin positively glow! And this glow does not depend on bronzer from a compact.

Recently, this beauty-from-within supplement was put to the test in a clinical study. Participants in this 16-week, double-blind, placebo-controlled, pilot study were randomized to either MSM (3 grams per day) or placebo, which was rice flour. Using instruments designed to analyze elasticity, hydration, firmness, and photographic measurements of wrinkles, those taking MSM had a measurable reduction in the number, size, and severity of facial wrinkles when compared to placebo. In particular, expert graders saw a significant improvement in crow's feet wrinkles in the MSM-treated group as compared to the placebo group.

The study also identified the effect that MSM had on genes associated with skin. Some of the skin aging genes that were positively modified by the MSM were the MMPs, the collagen-eating enzymes, genes associated with skin-barrier function (DSG3 and LCE3D), and aquaporin-3, a gene involved in skin hydration. This represents the theme of my book exactly: how to leverage epigenetics to modify our environment and improve how we age and how we look.

MSM is an inexpensive crystal powder that can be added to a glass of water, or added to a smoothie.

L-Carnosine, not to be confused with L-Carnitine, is another skin-beautifying supplement that is particularly important for vegans and vegetarians. It is a dipeptide, made up of two amino acids. L-Carnosine functions as an antioxidant, anti-inflammatory, *and* anti-glycation agent, making it a triple winner in the longevity department. L-Carnosine has been shown to both rejuvenate old cells and extend the functional life of skin's building blocks. L-Carnosine acts like a strong anti-glycation agent, preventing the crosslinking of collagen fibers in the skin that lead to wrinkling and sagging.

L-Carnosine is found in all of our body tissues, but unfortunately, levels decline with age. For a food source for L-carnosine, look no further than animal foods, especially beef, which is why vegetarians might want to consider supplementation.

Plants for Beauty

For millennia plants and their products have been used to preserve and enhance the beauty of skin. For most of history, that was all that was available to people. As people continue to explore non-surgical and less-invasive ways to preserve the way they age, plant products continue to have a place in the anti-aging arsenal.

Many of these ancient rituals now have the science behind them as to why they work. The Egyptian Queen Cleopatra, for example, was known for her milk and honey baths. Today we know that the milk contains lactic acid, an exfoliator still used today and, together, these ingredients softened and naturally exfoliated the skin while leaving a sweet smell behind. The desire for beauty is absolutely ancient and contemporary at the same time.

OPCs, Oligomeric Proanthocyanidins from grapeseed extract are a particular favorite that I like to recommend for skin. These phytonutrients from the polyphenol family have an amazing array of health benefits, many of which promote healthy skin. OPCs are anti-inflammatory and, remember, inflammation helps drive aging and wrinkles. OPCs also retard matrix metalloproteinases, those pesky enzymes that degrade the collagen and result in wrinkles. They have also shown positive effects in collagen strengthening, another plus for the aging facial structure.

OPCs have a near and dear place in my heart because they were the subject of my first published paper in a peer-reviewed medical journal. I became fascinated with them because they truly are multifunctional phyto powerhouses. OPCs are antibacterial, antiviral, anti-allergic, anticancer, increase microcirculation, and are good for the skin. This is quite an impressive package of goodies for one supplement.

Recent studies of OPCs from grapeseed extract have found them to mitigate the UV-radiation-induced oxidative stress in human skin that kicks off the inflammatory and collagen-degrading cascade that leads to wrinkles. It is always good to head this off at the top of the cascade.

As well, in a small group of Japanese women supplemented with orally administered grapeseed extract for 6 months, 83% of them had improvement in their chloasma, or facial hyperpigmentation that appears mask-like. Chloasma is a facial skin disorder involving too much melanin production that often plagues women and is very recalcitrant to various treatments. Sometimes it has been called the "mask of pregnancy" as it often occurs during that time.

The incidence of non-melanoma skin cancer has increased dramatically worldwide, accounting for more than 40% of all human cancers in the United States. Polyphenols found in a large variety of plant products, like grapeseed extract, have been found to be protective against UV-induced skin inflammation, proliferation, immunosuppression, DNA direct hits, and disruption of certain cellular signaling pathways; all steps leading to a diagnosis of squamous cell carcincoma and basal cell carcinoma, the non-melanoma skin cancers. As these forms of skin cancer continue to increase worldwide, it is necessary to study polyphenols like grapeseed proanthocyanidin complexes and evaluate them for their chemo-protective abilities.

Along those lines, grapeseed proanthocyanidins were found to turn on previously silenced tumor-suppressor genes in human skin cancer cells by epigenetic mechanisms. If we are able to turn the tumor-suppressor genes back on, we can better suppress the tumors. The loss of tumor-suppressor-gene activity is broadly implicated in most cancers, and a subject of much research. This is groundbreaking work that has significant implications for the epigenetic treatment and even prevention of skin cancers in humans.

Grapeseed extract has also demonstrated the ability to downregulate inflammation and immunosuppression brought on by UV-radiation exposure that potentially leads to skin cancer. Yes, you read that right; too much sunlight actually suppresses the immune system, while enough sunlight is necessary for proper immune function. Even Mother Nature loves moderation.

Beauty Boost

Grape Seed Extract

- Anti-inflammatory
- Reduces collagen breakdown
- Increases microcirculation
- Reduces hyperpigmentation

Resveratrol is a plant-derived polyphenol that has many antiaging activities making it a popular focus of longevity research today. It works against mitochondrial dysfunction and oxidative stress, two of the leading theories of aging. Mitochondria are the energy-making factories in all of your cells, and they make less energy as we age. Our cells use energy to do things like repair DNA, replace proteins and organelles, and take out the garbage (detox). Mitochondrial dysfunction is akin to if our body experienced an energy crisis: it is associated with virtually all degenerative diseases including Alzheimer's, type 2 diabetes, heart failure, and cancer. While perking up our mitochondria has already been thought of and done, actually finding a way to make more is newly discovered and is considered a boon in regenerative aging. Enter resveratrol.

Resveratrol is a naturally occurring polyphenol found in over 70 different species of plants, but the ones we most often hear about are grapes (red wine), cranberries, and peanuts. Resveratrol activates the SIRT1 genes which jumpstart the biochemical reactions leading to mitochondrial rejuvenation.

In a human study, a combination supplement of OPCs and resveratrol demonstrated the ability to resuscitate malingering mitochondria and make new ones. Mitochondria biogenesis (making new ones) is quite a hot topic in the longevity world, and resveratrol is one of the top supplements being investigated for its effect.

Resveratrol is considered a powerful antioxidant and Nrf-2 stimulator, with skin-enhancing properties. Resveratrol not only stops the free-radical cascade, but acts on a deeper level to stimulate our body's own production of downstream genes induced at the epigenetic level of mRNA and protein levels.

In a mouse study, resveratrol was shown to reverse skin atrophy, through its antioxidant capabilities and also its ability to rejuvenate mitochondria in the skin cells.

In another human study, a supplement containing resveratrol, ellagic acid, and OPCs was taken once per day for 60 days and compared against a control group who took a placebo. All parameters tested, including hydration, age spots, wrinkling, skin elasticity, roughness, and antioxidant markers in the skin, improved significantly as compared to the control group. This study illustrates the synergistic effect that can be achieved when certain phytonutrients are mixed together.

Curcumin is a polyphenol that accumulates in the rhizome of *Curcuma longa*, and is the most medicinally active compound in the popular spice, turmeric. It is commonly used in tasty curries and possesses several anti-aging mechanisms that can be employed for maintaining youthful looking skin. While curcumin has been used medicinally for thousands of years, modern science has recently begun to embrace it in a big way. Curcumin and ginger are in the same herb family and share many similar characteristics in terms of benefits to skin health.

In medicine, curcumin is strongly, almost miraculously, anti-inflammatory, antibacterial and antioxidant, and has shown benefits in cancer treatment and prevention, pain syndromes, type 2 diabetes, and cardiovascular health. In fact, curcumin is one of the most studied agents for cancer prevention and treatment with hundreds of articles published on its efficacy and mechanisms of action.

In terms of skin benefits, curcumin is a potent inhibitor of our inflammatory master switch, NF-kB, along with AP-1, a transcription factor also involved in switching on inflammation. In fact, curcumin is one of the star epigenetic gene modifiers because it can turn off the inflammation-induced wrinkle cascade and turn on your beauty genes instead! This has translated into help for skin diseases such as psoriasis, scleroderma, and vitiligo, and increases in wound healing.

Curcumin has also been studied for its ability to prevent skin cancer through suppression of inflammation and quenching of free radicals caused by solar radiation. It acts like a skin protector. In mice, both oral and topical application of curcumin have been shown to potently protect against UV-induced skin tumors.

Curcumin is a genius at turning off the wrinkle switch, but it turns out it is twice as helpful for skin since it turns on one of our beauty genes—Nrf-2. Nrf-2 is found in high amounts in the epidermis, the body's first contact point with the outside. This makes sense because your epidermis is always in contact with your environment and subject to environmental assault through sun, pollution, temperature changes, cigarette smoke, and the like. Nrf-2 is the skin's own defense mechanism against these exposures, and turns on the skin's own antioxidant and detoxifying enzymes in order to combat the noxious chemicals, or free radicals, before they can do damage to the skin cells that leads to aging and possibly skin cancer.

Let's talk more about the benefits of Nrf-2 (Nuclear factor-erythroid-2-related factor 2.) The discovery of Nrf-2 is a game changer in the whole anti-aging paradigm, even though the word is not out yet. It will soon throw the youth-seeking, rules-flaunting, baby boomers into a frenzy because Nrf-2 has emerged as the "guardian of health span and gatekeeper of species longevity," as one group of researchers coined it in 2010.

Nrf-2 is a transcription factor expressed in all tissues, some more than others, that stimulates the production of more than 200 different genes involved in cellular protection. Now that's a master switch! Could Nrf-2 be the "master switch" of aging?

Nrf-2 turns on your body's own production of antioxidants to quench free radicals, and also turns on your body's own detoxifying enzymes, such as glutathione and superoxide dismutase (SOD) that are used to detoxify toxins from food, pollutants, or even infections.

These two activities are powerful in terms of protecting your body from noxious aging agents; remember, your epidermis has high amounts of Nrf-2. During wound-healing, Nrf-2 is upregulated in your skin, and has also been found to be protective against UVB-induced skin cancer. Beautiful!

Nrf-2 also downregulates inflammation through multiple pathways, which has widespread implications for our overall health and prevention of disease, much or most of it due to chronic inflammation. And let's not forget that inflammation also is involved in skin aging, wrinkle formation, and loss of elasticity.

Beauty Boost

Nrf-2 (the Beauty Gene)

- Anti-inflammatory
- Antioxidant
- Detoxifying
- Protects skin against UV rays

Beauty Boosters

Nrf-2 (the Beauty Gene) Stimulators

Natural Substances	Found In
Curcumin	Tumeric
Carnosol	Rosemary
Quercetin	Onions, apples, kale
Resveratrol	Red wine, Polygonum cuspidatum, grapes
Sulphoraphane	Broccoli, cabbage, cruciferous veggies
Catechins	Green tea, chocolate

NF-kB Suppressors (the Wrinkle Master Switch)

Natural Substances	Found In
Curcumin	Tumeric
Quercetin	Onions, apples, kale
Resveratrol	Red wine, polygonum cuspidatum, grapes
Grape seed Extract (OPCs)	Supplement
EPA/DHA (Fish Oil)	Supplement
Vitamin C	Non-corn based preferred
Green Tea	Organic preferred

The science of skin aging has exploded over the last five or ten years and has now been defined right down to the molecular level. The study of genomics in aging skin provides multiple targets for preventing or slowing down the aging process in the skin. Through diet and lifestyle changes, including supplementation with certain targeted nutrients, we now have greater understanding, insight, and ability to exert some control over the aging process. The future of cosmetic medicine will be greatly enhanced by the concept of beauty from within and the adoption of lifestyle and diet strategies.

Applying the information

The Minimalist

- Add a high quality probiotic to your regimen
- Add grape seed extract, 100 mg per day.

The Middle Way: Accompanying the above,

- Add vitamin C 1,000 mg per day (non-corn source or camu camu powder)
- Astaxanthin 6 mg per day
- Fish oil 2 grams per day (if not on blood thinners)

The Beauty Buff: In Addition to All of the above,

- Curcumin (liposomal) 500 mg twice a day
- Resveratrol 200 mg per day (ideally trans-resveratrol from Polygonum cuspidum)

CHAPTER FIVE

Traveling for Beauty

"Sometimes your only available transportation is a leap of faith." — *Margaret Shepard*

TRAVELING CAN BE EXTREMELY HARD on your skin, particularly if you are traveling by air. Everyone has heard how dehydrating flying is, but there are proper steps to take to stay hydrated. IS there anything you can do to stay healthy while flying? This is your ultimate guide to staying healthy and beautiful while you are traveling.

Let's start with the hydration. Flying makes you lose more water by trans-epidermal water loss (TEWL). Obviously you must take in more water while you are flying. But those tiny cups of water that the flight attendants hand out sparingly are not even enough to stay properly hydrated on the ground! Always buy additional water to carry on the plane, and make sure you really hydrate before your flight. When the drinks cart comes around, request two cups of water at a time. This is in addition to drinking your own bottled water. Most people have experienced constipation when they travel. Believe it or not, dehydration (along with different food choices) is the culprit here. By snacking on cut-up vegetables and fruits that you bring from home, you also fill up on water since the water content is so high in them. Rest assured; you are also getting your fill of antioxidants that will help you resist the damaging free radicals to which you will be exposed.

Let me also mention that I find most people are dehydrated on a daily basis, and this has nothing to do with flying. Water is incredibly important for proper digestion, elimination, detoxification, and for your skin. Remember, skin is hydrated from within, from the water you drink. The general rule of thumb is to consume water at one-half your body weight in ounces, per day. If you exercise, or live in a very hot climate, drink more.

Alcohol is also dehydrating and, when you are in the air, it's even more so. If you are drinking alcohol during a flight, then you are NOT drinking water, thus intensifying the dehydration effects. Also, caffeinated beverages are dehydrating. The best beverage for flying and maintaining your skin's looks is water, hands down! If you are going to drink an alcoholic or caffeinated beverage, double up on your water intake to make up for the additional water loss.

For hydration that is externally applied, I recommend taking in a TSA-approved bag a small container of mineral water for spraying on your face. These are actually available to buy, but you can also just rebottle your own mineral water. Also, I recommend a rich, oil-based serum, like the Youth Serum from the IAMFINE® Pure Skin Collection (www.drannemariefine.com), and some cleanser; or even better, some of the new natural cleansing wipes that are out on the market and that you are allowed to use in your seat.

The day of your flight, wash your face as usual and apply your own serum or the IAMFINE® Youth Serum, 8-10 drops to your face. Massage in for about one minute. If you are using the IAMFINE® Youth Serum, add another drop to each nostril, just barely lubricating the inside of your nasal passage. The purpose of the Youth Serum applied to the inside tip of your nasal cavities is that the essential oils in the Youth Serum are antimicrobial and will help keep you healthy while you are flying, as well as prevent the nasal mucosa from getting too dried out.

Alternately, you can use plain vitamin E oil (or puncture a vitamin E capsule), one drop in each nostril to keep the nasal mucosa moist, which is what I used to do before I formulated the Youth Serum

The Youth Serum is a rich blend of organic seed oils that are specially formulated to deeply hydrate your skin, fight free radicals, the generation of which are ramped up when you fly, and address inflammation. The blend includes anti-aging essential oils sourced carefully from all over the world that are also antimicrobial and anti-inflammatory. By prepping your face with this nourishing anti-aging oil, you are protecting your face from dehydration (the oil is providing a barrier to TEWL), free radicals produced in abundance in flight, germs lurking everywhere on the airplane, and fighting the signs of aging all at once. Apply this Youth Serum, or layer a heavier-duty moisturizer of your own, over an antioxidant serum before flying to seal in the moisture you already have and inhibit the drying effects of cabin air.

If it is a flight longer than three hours, you can go into the lavatory and wash your face with cleanser, spray the mineral water, wait a few minutes while it dries, and then reapply the Youth Serum or the moisturizer of your choice. It is also nice to apply a few drops to the backs of your hands to keep them moisturized and protected. However, if you are using electronic devices like your computer on the flight, I wouldn't advise it. The oils on the hands are too messy.

I find it easier to fly without any makeup on because it is that much easier to keep misting with hydrating sprays, and applying and reapplying oil-based serums to keep the skin from drying out. Depending on your own skin hydration levels and length of your flight you can apply the serum every few hours. If you have a favorite balm, you can apply that to your nails and cuticles to keep them from drying out too.

Beauty has become more mobile friendly, so if you are inclined, you can even open a single use face or eye mask on your flight and apply for the specified time, and really enjoy a revitalizing facial experience that allows you to deplane with dewy fresh skin.

Beauty Boost

- No makeup on flight
- Antioxidant oil-based serum-apply every three hours or so
- Hydrate, hydrate, hydrate
- For extra special care, take along facial mask

Strategic use of supplements before, during, and after flying can greatly mitigate the biological stress of flying. One of the stressors of flying is the exposure to toxicants in the aircraft itself, such as flame retardants. Flame retardants have been found in 100% of dust samples from commercial aircraft, and in higher concentrations than have been found in commercial or residential environments. The reason is obvious: the foam that is found in airplane seats and other places is full of flame retardants in order to adhere to industry standards for retarding fire, an important consideration for a jet.

I will take a cocktail of supplements on my flights in order to counteract some of these environmental exposures. Before I fly, I make sure to take liposomal glutathione, a universal antioxidant and master detoxifier. If you don't have access to this, the glutathione precursor, N-acetyl-Cysteine can be taken. I also pre-load with vitamin C, grapeseed extract (for circulation), magnesium, Co-Q10, and certain immune boosting herbs. Midway through the flight I will take the same combination and, when I land, I will rehydrate with water and follow-up with a similar combination. While many people find they become ill after a flight, I have not found this to be a problem.

Another beauty robber encountered while flying is jet lag and other sleep disturbances. Lack of sleep will definitely make your skin look sallow and give you dark circles under your eyes. There are many techniques available for addressing these problems. One of them is, a few days before your trip, going to bed either a little later, or a little earlier, depending on the time zone to which you are traveling, which will help your body to adjust to the new schedule. This includes staying up if you land during the day even though it may be the middle of the night where you just left.

Another technique often mentioned is taking melatonin before bed when you arrive at your destination, as your pineal gland, the gland responsible for making melatonin in relationship to light entering the eye, is off schedule. This is also why it is recommended that you arrive in the daylight and make sure to expose your eyes to natural daylight at your new destination.

I frequently fly internationally for business and have found a far superior plan for combatting jet lag. My patients and I use Frequency Specific Microcurrent (FSM), an FDA-approved medical device, which I have programmed for jet lag. What is FSM? FSM is a noninvasive, biologic resonance inducer that affects tissues, organs, and the nervous system. The concept of **Biological Resonance** refers to all tissues having an ideal electrical frequency that coordinates physiological activity. When I program the unit for jet lag, I can target the pineal gland, which is responsible for secreting melatonin based on certain environmental clues, to reset, thus ameliorating the negative effects of landing in a different time zone than the one(s) just departed.

The portable FSM unit that I have been using in my practice for over ten years is an FDA-approved medical device that must be prescribed by a physician and then programmed for each individual. See the Resources section for how to obtain. Various protocols can be programmed and downloaded into the portable device making it easy and convenient for the patient to use as prescribed, even on an airplane. I make it a point to always travel with mine in my carry-on baggage.

The program for jet lag can be easily run in one's seat while actually flying through different time zones. This is my secret for international travel because I can hit the ground running, have a normal and productive day, right from the beginning of my trip. And because international travel is so long, I can run other programs from my seat such as one to rejuvenate the adrenals from the stress of traveling. I feel good when I travel!

Another way to literally ground yourself after traveling a long distance that involves no extra equipment at all, is to seek out nature upon arrival, to do something called earthing, and at the same time expose yourself to the natural sunlight which will help reestablish your circadian rhythms. The quicker you can reestablish your circadian rhythms in the new location, the faster your sleep, digestion, and brain functions will get back on track.

What is earthing? Earthing is simply contacting the earth with your bare feet. If you think about it, our ancestors spent most of their time in contact with the earth by wearing animal skin shoes and clothes, and even sleeping on animal skins—all natural materials. With the advent of plastics and insulating soles in our footwear instead of leather (a natural material), other synthetic materials, asphalt, and high-rise buildings, we no longer spend much time in contact with the earth.

The earth is electrically charged, as are we. In fact, the earth can be considered a giant reservoir of antioxidants, which are electron donors, due to its abundance of free electrons that flow into us when we contact the earth unimpeded by synthetic materials. Studies have shown that inflammation is reduced and wound healing improved, beginning with as little as 30 minutes of earthing. Could earthing, something that is free and easily accessible, be important for addressing our population's overall problem with chronic inflammation? This is a fascinating new perspective on health and aging that I anticipate will result in much further study and application.

For our purposes, upon landing, find a park or other natural area with grass, trees, sand, and even water. Beaches are great for earthing, but any ground works as long as it is not paved over in concrete and asphalt. Take off your shoes and put your bare feet on the earth. You can just sit there, or walk. The important thing is to have your bare feet contact the earth. In about 30-40 minutes you should begin feeling the energizing effects of earthing.

Even the busiest urban areas have parks, so getting back to nature should be easily accomplished. I am such a fan of earthing, that I have been known to hail a cab while traveling in a new place and simply stating, "Take me to the nearest beach or park" much to the consternation of the taxi driver who is used to being instructed as to a specific park or beach that the passenger wishes to see.

Try to reset your circadian rhythms by exposing yourself to natural daylight if it is day time, and avoid going to bed out of sync with your destination. Try to stay up until the sun goes down at least. Do not give in to naps upon arrival at your hotel, even though you may be tired. This is where earthing can be extremely helpful and bring a vibrancy and energy to your travels that you might not have even thought possible. Hydrate, hydrate, hydrate to make up for the dehydrating flight.

Digestion suffers with travel as well, resulting in constipation, indigestion, and appetite disturbances. Since we have already discussed the relationship between digestion and skin, it is wise to pay attention to this fact. The disturbance to circadian rhythm brought on by traveling through time zones also affects our digestion. Digestion is the last body system to get back on track as we change time zones. I recommend eating very lightly the day of travel to take the load off the digestive system.

What this means is take your own food. The quality of the processed, prepackaged, food-like substances masquerading as food is frightening. The refined grain content alone in the snacks and sandwiches provided on the flight is a nightmare for your digestive system, can produce wide blood sugar swings, and contains no fiber whatsoever, thus setting you up for constipation. As I am writing this, I am on a flight home from Ireland and the young woman in front of me just ordered, and paid for, a cylinder of Pringles to go with her soda. The sandwiches that were passed around were all white bread, completely devoid of any nutritional value or fiber whatsoever. The refined wheat flour, bleached and extruded into pretzel shapes, actually is considered a healthy snack!

Take your own food. While you cannot carry your own liquids from home, you can carry on your own snacks. I always carry on a large protein shake container that contains protein powder, chia seeds, and maca root—a wonderful combination to keep up endurance on a travel day. I also take nuts, goji berries, high-quality dark chocolate, and some high-quality, low-sugar, protein bars. Often I will make raw snacks at home and both carry them on board and pack them into my suitcase because they are chock full of real food with real nutrition.

Traveling in airplanes has also been associated with getting sick shortly after the flight. While many people feel this is due to the high percentage of recycled air on the flight, most infectious disease is transmitted by touching a contaminated surface. Some microbes can last about a week on surfaces, making a strong case for consistent hand washing with hot, soapy water in the restrooms, and using hand sanitizer in between. But beware of commercial hand sanitizers as they normally contain triclosan, a registered pesticide and antimicrobial chemical.

Triclosan, a broad spectrum antimicrobial agent, is found in common household products such as toothpaste, facewash, deodorant, many personal-care products such as hand sanitizers, and even mattresses, toothbrushes, and shoe insoles (to prevent bacterial odors). However, a U.S. FDA advisory committee has found that the household use of antibacterial products provides NO benefits whatsoever over good old plain soap and water and, now, the American Medical Association is even recommending that triclosan not be used in the home as it may add to the ongoing threat of bacterial resistance to antibiotics that we are already seeing. Recently the FDA banned the use of triclosan in soaps and body washes, but companies have some time to reformulate it out so it is still widely available.

Triclosan has been found in urine, plasma, and breast milk of humans. High levels of triclosan were found in 60% of human milk samples indicating its absorption potential. According to National Health and Nutrition Examination Survey (NHANES) data collected during 2003–2004, TCS was found in 75% of the analyzed urine samples, making this a fairly ubiquitous substance found in people.

There are non-toxic hand sanitizers available in the marketplace if you wish to augment your traditional hot water and soap handwashing. These typically contain essential oils which naturally contain antimicrobial compounds, which is why they are so widely used in natural medicine. I have seen lavender and lemon essential oil travel wipes available for the purpose of sanitizing hands while traveling. You can also use these natural hand sanitizing wipes to wipe down your tray table, armrests, and seat buckle in order to minimize your contact with all the microbes found lurking in these locations.

Noise on airplanes contributes to the overall stress levels. I didn't realize this until a few years ago when a colleague who travelled extensively reported that noise-cancelling headphones were worth their weight in gold. I received a pair as a gift and discovered that, while the noise cancelling effects were wonderful, they could also be used to listen to my own music, meditation tapes, and chanting playlists for further stress reduction. Since I cannot sleep at all on a flight, even an overnight flight, I wind up listening to soothing meditation-style tapes in order to at least travel in a more stress-reduced way.

Do travel with your essentials, including makeup must haves, toothbrush/toothpaste, and a change of clothes. This is just simple preparedness and makes your life easier in the case of lost or late luggage.

I once arrived in Paris for a speaking engagement and my luggage did not. I had never had the displeasure of losing my luggage and so I stayed at the baggage claim conveyor belt for a long, long time, hoping and wishing my bag would show up while simultaneously trying to process the idea that it would not. It did not, and then I was confronted with the sad realization that I would be speaking at a conference the very next day. There I was in my makeup-free, albeit adequately moisturized, face and yoga wear that doubled as leisure/travel wear, in tennis shoes, no less, with no travel bag of essentials. This was my grand experiment in traveling light (only a purse on board, no carry-on bag) and turned out to be an epic fail! Never travel without a carry-on bag that can get you through the next day if your luggage does not arrive.

I exited the taxi and marched straight to the Sephora on the Champs-Elysees and reached them before they even opened for the day. At this Sephora, standard opening procedure consisted of all the salespeople lining up on both sides of the doors as the doors open in the morning, and then they all clap their hands as the cosmetically deprived are ushered in to the deafening roar of rock music. As I moved through the line of salespeople, one saleswoman near the end took one look at me and took me by the hand to her chair, shaking her head sadly. In lieu of speaking French, I haplessly tried to mime that I had a speaking engagement the next day and needed to look presentable but also professional. She deftly sized me up and began applying a dizzying array of skin-care and cosmetic products to my face. I bought nearly every product, including the skin-care products because I had none with me. And then I was off to purchase an entire outfit for my presentation.

All of this is avoidable if you travel with your makeup and skin-care essentials, all in TSA approved containers, of course. Most skin care and makeup lines now have travel kits that sport smaller sized versions of their full-sized products that can be easily put in your overnight bag.

Do not forget the sunscreen. Many who are traveling will spend more time outdoors than normal and this means you will be exposing your skin to more sun. A sunburn on vacation can really complicate your stay and wreak havoc on your skin. And don't forget, traveling in a car does not protect you against the sun's rays.

I like to keep my energy high while traveling so I can really enjoy new vistas and experiences. It is too easy to fall out of sync with our normal routines while traveling and then experience lower energy, poorer sleep, and other health consequences. Who wants to be tired when traveling?

One important strategy to keep your energy high is to keep up your exercise and yoga routines. Traveling involves a lot of sitting, which leads to poor circulation, muscle stiffness, and lack of energy. I typically get in some yoga stretches at the airport prior to boarding, even though it is hardly the right venue. Stand up and stretch, walk to the restrooms, do seated exercises while you are on the airplane. If you are traveling by train you may have more opportunity to walk around.

Once you arrive at your destination, make sure to work in some exercise. If your hotel has a gym, it is pretty easy to schedule in some time for movement. If you don't like gyms, be sure to get outside and walk, or run, or find a local venue for your activity of choice. It is sure a lot easier now to exercise on the road than it was even 10 years ago. If you are completely stuck, remember that jogging in place in your hotel room and doing sit-ups, pushups, and burpees will all get your heart rate up. Or just put on some music and dance, either in the privacy of your own hotel room or out on a dance floor.

Keeping up your muscle strength, cardiovascular fitness, and flexibility all go a long way to keeping your energy and mood high. A strong body; now that makes you feel more beautiful!

By following some of the advice above you will land at your destination and embark like a radiant diva ready to take on the world.

Applying the information

The Minimalist

- No alcohol on flight; lots and lots of water
- Eat lightly, preferably with high-quality snacks that you brought from home

The Middle Way: Accompanying the above,

- Apply IAMFINE® Youth Serum to your face and nostrils before you fly, reapply as needed

The Beauty Buff: In Addition to All of the above,

- Pre-load with glutathione or N-acetyl-Cysteine, Grapeseed Extract, and vitamin C, magnesium, and Co-Q10
- Re-dose every 3 hours on longer flights
- Invest in a Frequency Specific Microcurrent unit so that you can treat yourself for jet lag and any other health issues, such as digestive or adrenal health, while you are flying: see Resources

CHAPTER SIX

Detoxification for Beauty

"Toxicity is at the root of most chronic disease, including skin diseases."- Dr. Fine

Organs of Elimination

WHAT MOST BEAUTY EXPERTS cannot tell you is that a beautiful face and glowing skin depend primarily on the health of your digestive and elimination systems—the body's built-in system to get rid of wastes and toxins. THIS is probably the greatest secret to having beautiful, clear, and healthy skin. And yet, most skin-care products and advice focus solely on targeting the skin from the outside. This is completely backwards.

Believe it or not, your skin is actually the body's largest organ of elimination. Your desire to be beautiful is actually dependent on your commitment to your overall health and vitality, and having functional organs of elimination is a requirement of both. As I have said before, clear, radiant skin is simply a reflection of your underlying good health. The healthiest and most beautiful skin is apparent when the body's detoxification process is working and toxins can be eliminated through the digestive tract, kidneys, and lungs.

The organs of elimination are lungs, colon, liver, kidneys, and skin. These are the pathways that rid your body of toxins that have been either produced internally through the regular metabolism of the body or acquired from outside toxins that have been ingested, absorbed through the skin, or inhaled. If the organs of elimination are not open, for example, if constipation, indigestion, insufficient water intake, or lack of sweating occurs, the skin will take up the slack and discharges will show up on the skin as spots or acne, rashes, dull or dry skin, or discoloration.

The liver is the primary detoxification organ in the body as it filters blood coming directly from the intestines and prepares, through three phases, toxins for elimination from the body. It should not be surprising that there is a strong relationship between the health of the liver and the rest of the digestive system, and the health and appearance of the skin. If the liver or colon is sluggish or overwhelmed, the toxins will have to be eliminated through the skin because the primary routes of detoxification are not working at their optimal levels.

Even when the other organs of elimination are open, the skin regularly removes wastes from the body through sweating and shedding of old, dead skin cells. In fact, your skin performs most of these detoxification processes overnight while you sleep; another reasons why it is called Beauty Sleep! When you don't get your beauty sleep, your skin shows the telltale signs: dark circles under the eyes, loss of radiance, more lines, and wrinkles.

In our Westernized society, the organs of elimination are under more pressure now than ever, and little thought is given to their function, let alone maintenance and health. While our excretory systems worked well for our ancient ancestors who lived in a more pristine, pre-industrial and primitive culture, it is having a hard time keeping up with the 80,000-plus registered chemicals currently in use in our world today.

As someone who has a genetic predisposition to poor detoxification, I was drawn to this area because, by using certain detoxification protocols and enhancing my detoxification enzyme system, I was finally able to overcome my genetic obstacles to detox and overcome my health challenges. In naturopathic medicine, we seek to find the root cause of illness, not just cover it up with a drug or cut out the offending part. Much to my astonishment, my underlying inability to excrete toxins was the ultimate cause of my medical problems. In fact, toxicity is at the root of most chronic disease and this is why I focus on environmental medicine.

Pollution and Your Skin

Body burden refers to the total amount of toxins and chemicals that accumulate in our bodies, starting even before we are born. Every day we are exposed to toxins from our food and water supply, air pollution, heavy metals, pesticides, plastics, aldehydes, drugs, flame retardants, formaldehyde, PCBs (polychlorinated biphenyls), and certain ingredients from personal-care products. Many of these substances are fat-soluble, so they accumulate in our fatty tissues including our endocrine system, which includes our thyroid, adrenal, pituitary, testes and ovaries, and our brain, which is mostly fat.

What's even more disturbing is that babies are being born now "pre-polluted." A landmark study published in 2005 found nearly 300 different toxicants in newborn babies' umbilical cord blood. Not too long ago, it was felt that the placenta protected the fetus from pollutants, but now it is known that the umbilical cord provides a continuous flow of blood from mom that also contains the same pollutants that mom has in her body, including pesticides, certain ingredients from personal-care products, and waste from the burning of fossil fuels.

Interestingly, the CDC (Center for Disease Control) has been studying and quantifying the body burden in humans for many years. Every few years, they publish the National Report on Human Exposure to Environmental Chemicals where they describe what chemicals they are testing for in the current report, and then provide quantitative data referring to the amounts found in Americans.

Our skin is constantly and directly exposed to environmental insults like cigarette smoke, pollution, excess sun exposure, and mechanical and chemical effects that result in increased free-radical formation that can exceed our innate ability to quench, leading to premature aging of the skin. The effects of smoking on premature aging of the skin are well known, but accumulating scientific evidence now points to air pollution's role in extrinsic aging.

Ambient particulate matter from traffic exhaust has been shown to prematurely age the skin in several studies. Most significantly, traffic exhaust increases those dreaded age spots on the skin—one of the most visible signs of aging skin. Women living in big cities were found to have prematurely aged skin compared to women living in less urban areas. Until very recently, it was believed that age spots and other forms of hyperpigmentation resulted primarily from sun exposure. As worldwide air pollution is a major health concern, it is important to factor the air-pollution factor into our skin-care protocols and considerations.

The very components in our skin, such as collagen and elastin, that maintain our cellular structure and integrity, are changed when exposed to particulate matter and other elements of pollution. Collagen alone constitutes about 70% of the weight of skin and provides the mechanical strength and structural support to the skin. When these components are degraded as a result of exposure to sun and pollution, sagging, dryness, and wrinkling result. Additionally, the skin's ability to detoxify is damaged, leading to further aging.

For these reasons, expect to see a surge in anti-pollution skin-care products being brought to market in the near future. In Asia, which continues to have high levels of air pollution, the global market research firm, Mintel, reports that this category—the anti-pollution category—is the one to watch, with new products growing at 63% from 2011 to 2013.

This is why I am a big fan of anti-pollution masks. I recommend using one per week for women over forty, and twice weekly for younger women who have more oil in their skin. As a category, facial masks continue to grow and expand their reach and stated skin goals. I recommend a mask made with calcium bentonite clay that strongly absorbs toxins through the skin, draws blood flow up to the outer surface of the skin (epidermis), and tightens as it does so. The

IAMFINE® Purifying Mask is one such mask and is available at www.drannemariefine.com

---

Beauty Boost

Steps to Protect Against Environmental Insults

- Wear a physical sunblock on your face and hands (not sunscreen)
- Wear a hat when outside
- Consume liberal amounts of plant foods for their antioxidants
- Wear moisturizer as it helps protect your skin's barrier function
- Wash face twice daily to remove makeup and pollution
- Use a facial mask once a week to deep clean
- Apply topical antioxidant serums

The Liver

The Three Phases of Detoxification

The liver detoxifies through three processes, Phase I, Phase II, and Phase III. In Phase I, the group of enzymes known as cytochrome P450 begins the process by making the toxins more water soluble. Water-soluble toxins are more easily excreted, but many of the toxins that we are taking into our bodies are fat-soluble, which means they are preferentially stored in our fatty tissues rather than excreted in our urine. In Phase II, further modification of the water-soluble toxins is performed and the toxin intermediates are also rendered less toxic. In Phase III, the new compounds are removed from the cell and begin the journey to excretion from the body through bowels, kidneys, or skin.

Phase I and Phase II also need to work in sync with each other, otherwise the resulting reactive intermediaries may become more dangerous than the original toxins. The intermediates from Phase I need to be promptly and efficiently moved into Phase II to minimize their deleterious impact on the body. This can be achieved through proper nutrition and supplementation.

Increased Phase I without a resulting increase in Phase II detoxification activity can be caused by tobacco smoke, high alcohol intake, ingestion of standard vegetable oils, and consuming charbroiled meats. If Phase I is overactive, then Phase II will have a buildup of reactive intermediates that, in turn, can result in tissue damage and disease.

Individuals who have this imbalance between Phase I and Phase II typically exhibit high sensitivity to fumes (scented products), react poorly to various pharmaceutical drugs by experiencing all or many of the side effects or reduced clearance of them, and have problems clearing caffeine from their system. These are very sensitive people who often don't understand why they have so much difficulty with their environment.

When Phase III detoxification is impaired, the toxins will be forced to be excreted from the skin. This can manifest in skin rashes and blemishes. Constipation can also result in skin blemishes, as the toxins that are in line for excretion are stalled and reabsorbed into the blood stream, only to find their way out of the body on the surface of your skin.

Every toxin and even hormones and other products that your body makes internally have to go to the liver to be processed this way into a more easily excreted form that can then be expelled through the colon. An overworked liver means that it is unable to keep up with the steady flow of toxins that it receives. One of the first signs that the liver is congested is bowel problems such as constipation. Constipation is a problem because the colon reabsorbs toxins if the transit time is slowed and the waste is backed up. This means that you are essentially getting double the dose of toxins; first when they enter your body, and then when they are reabsorbed into the bloodstream from the colon and recirculated throughout the body. Have you ever noticed that when you are constipated, you often experience a headache? That is one effect of the reabsorption of toxins from your stalled colon.

Other symptoms of a sluggish liver include:

- Headaches/migraines
- Acne/skin rashes
- Brain fog
- Poor tolerance to cleaning chemicals, fragrances, coffee, and alcohol
- Premenstrual syndrome
- Constipation
- Chronic fatigue
- Unexplained nausea
- Body odor

The reason why people who finish a detoxification program have glowing skin is because they have just greatly eliminated a lot of toxins from their body. Supporting your liver will have very positive effects on your skin.

The Best Liver Cleansing Foods

- Artichokes
- Beets
- Lemons
- Parsley
- Garlic
- Dandelion greens
- Burdock root
- Cruciferous vegetables

Artichokes are one of the world's oldest plants and medicines. The pharmacological effects of artichokes were known back in the seventeenth century, and were confirmed in recent studies to be stimulating on the liver and gallbladder, thus providing support for detoxification. Extensive herbal and biomedical research has concluded that the artichoke is liver protective, induces bile, and lowers cholesterol.

Lemons are an important medicinal food that lends itself to many applications. Their key actions are as antiseptic, antibacterial, antioxidant, and they also have a tonic effect on the liver. Lemons are high in vitamin C, which is important and necessary for collagen formation, and potassium which is good for energy, skin, and nerves. They are also very alkaline.

One simple way to introduce a detoxifying drink into your morning routine is to drink warm lemon water. Warm lemon water is known for its ability to directly stimulate and detoxify the liver and even stimulate a bowel movement.

It is crucial to make this lemon water at home and not rely on store bought lemon juices that are often loaded with sugar, have depleted nutrient levels, and are pasteurized, which will simply not offer the same benefits. Use organic lemons if possible; if you have access to fresh lemons from a tree of your own (or a friend's) that is best. Squeeze one-half to a whole lemon into one glass of pure, warm water. Consume the entire glass each morning before breakfast.

Beets are classic for liver cleansing. They are rich in folates, phosphorus, vitamin C, copper, potassium, and manganese. Beets also contain betaine and the phytonutrient betalains, which are used in phase II liver detoxification processes. Beets are best when juiced, and you must begin with small amounts as they are very detoxifying. One side effect when juicing beets is that you may experience some redness in your urine or stool. This is from the red pigment in the beets themselves.

One of parsley's volatile oils—myristicin—has been shown to activate the enzyme *glutathione-S-transferase*, which helps attach the molecule glutathione to oxidized molecules that would otherwise do damage in the body. This is how it aids in detoxification. The flavonoids in parsley—especially luteolin—have been shown to function as antioxidants that combine with highly reactive oxygen-containing molecules (called oxygen radicals) and help prevent oxygen-based damage to cells

Garlic is a potent detox favorite, rife with sulfur compounds that are crucial to making compounds such as glutathione, one of the body's top antioxidants and detoxifying agents. Garlic can be juiced. Garlic also has many immune stimulating properties, which is why, when I feel a cold coming on, I add several cloves to my juice or make a raw garlic sandwich, which is simply raw garlic chopped and left to sit for a few minutes, put between buttered bread.

Dandelion greens, those eyesores of old, are secret agents of detoxification. The bitter compounds in dandelion leaves and root help stimulate digestion and are mild laxatives. They also increase bile production in the gall bladder and bile flow from the liver. In some cultures, salads featuring fresh dandelion greens are eaten in the spring as part of a seasonal cleanse.

Burdock root has been used traditionally in ancient healing systems to alleviate skin challenges such as rashes, acne, abscesses, local skin infections, eczema, and psoriasis. In Ayurvedic medicine, burdock root is considered a blood purifier and skin cleanser. Burdock root is especially valuable when taken a few days prior to menstruation to prevent hormonally driven acne.

→ Cauliflower, broc, Bok Choy Cabbage, brussels

Cruciferous vegetables are an entire family of vegetables known for their distinctive group of phytonutrients called glucosinolates, which are able to upregulate liver detoxification enzymes. So far, 100 unique glucosinolates have been identified by scientists. Sulphoraphane is one that has received much attention and research studies. It is associated with induction of Nrf-2, our Master Switch, which is responsible for upregulating the body's antioxidant response and phase II liver enzymes.

All of us have variations in our detoxification enzyme systems called single nucleotide polymorphisms (SNPs). Some enzymes work slower in some people than in others; some enzymes work faster in some people than in others. This is all part of our biochemical individuality and the reason why the same diet, or supplement, or the same drugs don't work the same in everyone. Foods and phytonutrients have the ability to affect these enzymes. These SNPs can be tested through specialized labs and offer great insight into one's detoxification abilities.

Cruciferous vegetables are a family of vegetables that have many SNP modifying phytonutrients. This is why they are so powerful at supporting detoxification.

Cruciferous Vegetables

- Arugula
- Bok choy
- Broccoli
- Brussels sprouts
- Cabbage
- Cauliflower
- Chinese cabbage
- Collard greens
- Daikon radish
- Horseradish
- Kale
- Kohlrabi
- Land cress
- Mustard greens
- Radish
- Rutabaga
- Shepherd's purse
- Turnip
- Watercress

Dry Skin Brushing

One of the great benefits to having our largest organ on the outside of our body is that we can utilize it very easily. Our skin serves as a direct link to our other organs and can be easily accessed to either nourish or detoxify our body. On the flip side, we also absorb more impurities through our skin than any other organ in our bodies. This is simply not adequately addressed enough, but is one of the reasons I am so passionate about using non-toxic skin-care products and care in deciding which fabrics to let next to my skin.

The ability of the skin to absorb substances is already known. We use transdermal patches for certain medications, a hot Epsom salts bath relaxes our muscles, and a drop of essential oil placed on the foot will travel to the head about 10 minutes later.

The skin's ability to excrete toxins, however, is not as well emphasized. The skin is sometimes referred to as the third lung or the third kidney. Up to two pounds of waste are eliminated every day through our skin. This is why the skin is often the very first place an imbalance in the body may appear as the skin tries desperately to eliminate waste. Eruptions, blemishes, rashes, odors, and even colors may appear.

The age-old practice of daily skin brushing is a method of aiding the skin in this detoxifying process. Skin brushing, when performed daily and consistently, is a marvelous aid in having soft, beautiful, and blemish-free skin all over your body, not just on your face. It is easy to do, requires minimal investment, and feels good too.

The substances that have been analyzed that fall off the body during skin brushing are not only dead skin cells, which we would expect, but discharges, urea, sodium chloride, sebum, and metabolic wastes.

Dry skin brushing also addresses the lymphatic system which is essential to removing wastes throughout the body. Indeed, that is its function. And yet, unlike our circulatory system, there is no pump (the heart) to keep the fluid moving. Your lymphatic system moves through the body picking up waste and excretes it through the skin, kidneys, and other organs of elimination. Do you have trouble with cellulite? Cellulite is a condition of trapped toxins underneath the skin that is greatly helped by proper lymphatic circulation.

Exercise is one way to get the lymph moving. But as we'll see, daily skin brushing does as well by jumpstarting the lymphatic drainage system, which allows wastes to be excreted regularly through the skin.

Beauty Boost

Dry Skin Brushing Benefits:

- Tightens skin
- Exfoliates top layer of dead skin cells, revealing newer, radiant skin
- Cleanses lymph system
- Helps with cellulite
- Strengthens the immune system
- Stimulates circulation
- Results in softer skin

Directions for Dry Skin Brushing

- Buy a long handled natural bristle brush (available at health food stores).

- Brush skin while it is dry, this means before your shower.
- Always brush towards the heart.
- Start with your feet, on your soles, brush next your ankles, calves and thighs using light upward strokes.
- Brush upwards on your stomach and buttocks, always sweeping towards the heart.
- Start on the back of the hands and brush to shoulders.
- Lightly brush the neck in a downward direction.
- Take a shower.

Sauna

One of the mainstays of detoxification is sauna therapy. Saunas have been used for hundreds of years in various cultures to promote health via sweating. In the Scandinavian countries, for example, inhabitants typically will have a sauna in the home and it is used at least weekly by the whole family for health promotion. In other cultures, such as Native Americans, this took the form of the sweat lodge ceremony, where intense sweating was accompanied by spiritual cleansing as well.

How does a sauna detoxify from a physiological standpoint? Saunas produce thermal stress or load to the body that initiates an autonomic nervous system response that increases peripheral circulation from 5-10% of cardiac output to a maximum of 60-70%. This results in perspiration, with some people being able to excrete nearly 2 liters per hour. As sweat is a primary route of excretion of toxins from the body, sauna therapy is recognized as a safe and effective way to promote and maintain health.

The increase in circulation also brings more oxygen and nutrients to tissues, while also carrying away wastes. Documented substances found in sweat from people undergoing sauna therapy include toxic heavy metals such as cadmium, nickel, lead, and aluminum, uranium, solvents, polychlorinated biphenyls (PCBs), bisphenol A, and phthalates. The last two substances are found in many common personal-care products and are considered hormone disruptors.

As far as the skin goes, the increased circulation, perfusion of oxygen and nutrients, and elimination of sweat and toxins provide many benefits to the skin. Most of my patients report smoother, softer skin after beginning a sauna protocol. Sauna is particularly good for psoriasis, a skin condition that is difficult to treat, and eczema, which is very common. A study published in *Dermatology* reported that sauna therapy was found to result in a more stable epidermal-barrier function and an increase in stratum corneum hydration. Skin epidermal-barrier function is critically important to our skin at any age, and the breakdown of this barrier for any reason causes problems such as rashes, eruptions, dry skin, and poor wound healing.

As a bonus, infrared sauna has been shown to increase collagen and elastin by stimulating skin cells. In one study of women, a six-month sauna period produced improvements in roughness and tightness, skin color, tone, and wrinkles. However, no improvement was noted in age spots.

Regular use of a sauna is a health-promoting therapy that not only rids us of our continually increasing load of toxicants in our body, but is also relaxing, reduces blood pressure, oxygenates our tissues, reduces pain and muscle stiffness, and can improve our skin's appearance. I believe a sauna is a must for every home.

Supporting Detoxification and Colon Health

It is exceedingly trendy today to see marketing schemes touting the amazing benefits of "detoxes" or "cleanses." When it comes to detoxification and "cleanses," there is no need to embark upon costly and sugar-ridden juice "cleanses" or colon-cleansing products from the health-food store, or even water fasting. The liver actually requires protein in order to do its detoxification work, so food and protein are required, and not eating might liberate some toxins from your fat cell, but then they will simply recirculate in your body.

Another important consideration is that a three-day "cleanse" will have next to no impact on your years' and decade's worth of exposure to ongoing environmental toxicants or total body burden. Detoxification that makes a difference needs to be incorporated into your lifestyle for a longer period of time, and repeated as your *exposure to these environmental toxicants occurs on a daily basis every day of your life.* In fact, I incorporate detoxification strategies into every day of my life in order to keep up with the sheer volume of chemical exposures in my life.

Designing a detoxification protocol involving certain foods and supplements and depuration protocols is a complex endeavor that, ideally, would involve your naturopathic physician or other integrative healthcare provider who can take a medical history, an environmental exposure history, and order the appropriate testing .This way, a personalized plan can be developed for you that would result in the most effective and safe protocol. For a list of doctors who have additional training in environmental medicine see www.naturopathicenvironment.com.

However, there are definitely guidelines for embracing a detoxification lifestyle. A whole foods, fresh, organic, and unprocessed diet is key for saturating the body with the nutrients and phytochemicals necessary for supporting proper detoxification. Emphasize vegetables, especially green leafy vegetables and cruciferous vegetables. Eat organic to reduce your exposure to pesticides and herbicides. Drink plenty of water (the liver also needs water in order to do its job of detoxification). Minimize or completely cut out caffeine, sugar, and alcohol.

For a more extensive discussion of environmental toxins and how to avoid them and institute daily detoxification steps, see my Daily Detox for Living in a Toxic Soup video here:

https://vimeo.com/197836986

Don't forget to sweat, either from sauna or regular exercise. Sweating is one of the secrets to getting the glow! I have had a sauna in my home for over 10 years and I use it regularly.

Applying the information

The Minimalist

- **Go organic.** This is an easy choice, once you become aware that to buy conventional means voluntarily exposing yourself and your family to pesticides, herbicides, and fungicides. If you are not going to buy all organic, see https://www.ewg.org/foodnews/ for a list of the foods most and least likely to have pesticide residues.

The Middle Way: Accompanying the above,

- Add dry skin brushing and 3-5 more servings per day of cruciferous vegetables from the list above.

The Beauty Buff: In Addition to All of the above,

- Schedule a consultation with a naturopathic or integrative doctor trained in Environmental Medicine who can properly assess and design a personalized detoxification protocol for you. www.naturopathicenvironment.com lists them.

CHAPTER SEVEN

Emotional Well-Being
for Beauty

"Beauty is not in the face; beauty is a light in the heart."—**Kahlil Gibran**

NOWHERE IN THE BODY does the mind-body connection have such a profound and visible effect than on the skin. The skin acts like a barometer, reflecting to the world your current emotional state. You may be wearing your heart and your mind on your face! Think about what you are feeling when you blush or how your face looks when you are angry. Recall the last time you were under a lot of pressure and stress and your face broke out, usually right before an important social occasion. This is because there is a robust neuro-endocrine-skin connection, which means your brain and your skin are communicating all the time.

The origin of this fascinating connection is rooted in the fact that our skin and our nervous system derive from the same embryonic germline. Our skin cells actually express the same proteins that our nervous system does. Our emotional states directly affect our skin and the rest of our body. It is not possible to delineate the mind and the body as they are completely intertwined. This is an important fact to remember when encountering any health challenge. Let's make it work for us. Because our mental and emotional states can help us age more gracefully, or accelerate our aging, we get to choose.

Stress

Psychological stress upregulates the nervous system, which results in formation of free radicals, immune dysfunction, and DNA damage—all of which can result in skin-related decline in collagen and elastin and the formation of wrinkles and furrows. Stress also increases our adrenal output of cortisol, our major stress hormone, which breaks down our muscle tissue, thins our skin, breaks down our bones, keeps us from getting our beauty sleep, and elevates blood sugar. Excess cortisol is one of our prime aging mechanisms. Now you know why stress reduction is so important to creating a happy and healthy life.

By way of contrast, emotional states of peace, joy, gratitude, and compassion have been found to lower stress levels. Meditation and mindfulness practices have been shown time and time again in the literature to directly lower cortisol levels and reduce oxidative stress, and even protect against short telomeres (another biological marker of aging), all factors in maintaining our lovely skin well into our later years.

Poor stress management and coping skills have been found to accelerate aging and a host of other chronic diseases, leading to increasing study of stress management techniques as solutions.

Meditation and mindfulness-based meditation practices, or Mindfulness Based Stress Reduction (MGSR), have become increasingly popular and have been shown to benefit psychological, neurological, endocrine, and immune factors. What we are learning is that these benefits can lead to more youthful aging *and* better health.

While stress and premature aging have been linked, what about other less-than-desirable emotions, such as anxiety and depression? Are they pro-aging as well?

A very large, Danish, twins study involving 1,800 twins in their seventies looked at environmental factors in perceived facial aging in an attempt to answer the question, "Why do some people look better than their chronological age, and why do some people look worse?"

Twin studies are often used to tease out the effect of nature (genes) versus nurture (environment) on health outcomes. Twin studies are fascinating because they demonstrate how much our environment really affects us. If it were "all in the genes," identical twins would have all the same health outcomes and, clearly, they do not. Most twin studies do not show a 100% correlation between twins and their health issues, which allows scientists to focus on the effect of environment.

In one particular twin study it was confirmed that sun and smoking are two strong factors that made people look older than their age. However, it also highlighted some interesting connections between mental health status and skin aging; namely, that a higher score in depressive symptoms in one twin was associated with a more visually aged face. In women, this fact accounted for almost five years of additional age.

Furthermore, a lower socioeconomic reality was also associated with greater perceived age. In this group, chronic stress, anxiety, depression, and even a greater physical workload were all higher. It is not hard to imagine that the subjects in the higher socioeconomic group enjoyed greater financial security, less stress, and more disposable income with which to purchase healthier foods, along with all those classes in yoga, mindfulness, and the gym membership.

Stress is linked to virtually every disease imaginable, if not as a trigger, then as an exacerbating factor. Stress is one of the main epigenetic factors that play into the genetic expression of our skin. Stress has been linked to acne, atopic dermatitis, psoriasis, even skin cancer. Our stress response, which for millennia was only activated very occasionally and was perfectly designed to shunt blood from unnecessary activities such as digesting food to the extremities (your last meal doesn't need to be digested if you must run to avoid becoming the wooly mammoth's latest meal), speed up the heart, and quicken all senses, all through a squirt of epinephrine and cortisol from the adrenal glands, now is activated multiple times per day. Our nervous system was never designed to be this active.

In today's highly stressed society, we have added mobile technology and are constantly connected to our work, our family, and our friends. It is next to impossible to truly get away from it all. Many people even go on vacation bringing their many devices with them, and then are not able to really let go and relax because they have not unplugged from the world. Many people report that when they get back from vacation they need another vacation to recover! Our pace and all the things on our to-do lists have become relentless. We are bombarded with more information in a day than we used to get over a period of months or even years. We are on information overload and it is showing up in elevated stress levels in many people.

We often even begin our day with a spike in stress hormones. The loud, obnoxious buzzer from your alarm clock can also jolt your adrenals to spike cortisol. I don't think that is a good way to start your day, with a huge burst of stress hormones. Years ago, I purchased a "Zen" alarm clock that begins 20 minutes before wake-up time to emit more light, to simulate the fact that, for thousands of years, we went to bed when the sun went down, and woke up when the sun came up. Then, at wake-up time a soft chime ensues, getting louder slowly as it repeats at increasingly shorter intervals until, voila! I have regained consciousness without being startled awake. This is a gentler way to wake up without alarming your adrenal glands that a crisis is in progress right now and you need to leap out of bed immediately to put out the fire.

Just beginning a work day by turning on your computer can be stressful, as the moment you turn it on you may have 100 emails already vying for your attention.

Chronic stress results in chronically elevated levels of a stress hormone called cortisol. While estrogen, progesterone, and testosterone get a lot of press in relation to aging, cortisol is involved as well. Cortisol is essential for life, but when it is chronically elevated, it is associated with inflammation, increased oxidative stress, and degrades the collagen in our skin by turning on the MMPs (matrix metalloproteinases) that break down collagen. So, the damaging effects of stress can be viewed as epigenetically altering the normal rate of aging in our skin by concurrently destroying existing collagen and decreasing new collagen formation. Fortunately there are ways to decrease stress, which we will discuss later in this chapter.

An important point here is that stress involves perception of stress. It is really the stress *response* that gets us into trouble here and not the actual event or, in many cases, an anticipated event which never comes to pass. We have a choice on how we react to potentially stressful situations. People perceive the same stressful or traumatic event differently. A study elegantly demonstrated this by showing that women with the highest levels of *perceived* stress actually had cellular markers of longevity much reduced from the women with the least *perceived* stress in their lives.

The idea of stress perception can also be illustrated in another one of the leading theories of aging, which is that the protective ends of our DNA (called telomeres) shorten as we age. Elizabeth Blackburn, PhD, who discovered telomeres and won a Nobel Prize for doing so, explained that, ultimately, they become so short that the end of our DNA unravels and we can no longer replicate our cells, so they die. Remarkably, mental and emotional stress produces a more rapid shortening of the telomeres—and leads to faster aging.

For example, in one study of caregivers of sick patients, the health of the caregivers' telomeres was determined by their attitude. It sounds impossible, but it's true. The caregivers who felt that the ongoing care was a heavy burden had shorter telomeres, while those who saw their work as a blessing and even an opportunity to be generous and compassionate had no shortening. **Stress involves perception of stress.** The same event can provoke entirely different emotional states in different people, even in the same family.

Stress directly affects your genes. One of the strongest epigenetic influencers of genetic expression is *stress*, along with diet, environmental toxicant exposure, lifestyle, thoughts, and beliefs. All of these epigenetic influences can be modified to some extent, and addressing stress can yield not only more radiant, healthy skin, but better health, longevity, and wellbeing throughout the entire mind and body.

By now it is clear, stress influences nearly every step in the cascade of wrinkle formation. Chronic stress, anxiety, and depression all increase the production of free radicals, which sit at the top of the cascade as one of the primary drivers of skin aging. Stress also increases the inflammatory chemicals which promote wrinkling and feed back into the free-radical pathway, culminating in skin aging.

One aspect of psychological stress and anxiety that we have not covered yet is its effect on the barrier function of the skin. One skin function is to provide the barrier; to protect the body from microbial invaders and regulate water evaporation—in essence, not letting the skin dry out. Stress has been shown to compromise this barrier by increasing trans-epidermal water loss (TEWL) resulting in dry, rough, and scaly skin. One might even say that stress can cause a nervous breakdown of the skin, since that is literally what is happening! One study that examined this demonstrated that this disruption in skin-barrier function from stress is also associated with blood levels of inflammatory chemicals. And we know that inflammation drives wrinkle formation too.

I really love the study that was done that used humor to heal the skin. Specifically, a humorous movie was shown to a group of elderly patients with atopic dermatitis, an inflammatory skin condition. The same funny movie was shown to a control group who did not have the skin condition. Both groups demonstrated reduced skin water loss and increased serum testosterone levels after watching the movie every night for two weeks. Both groups benefitted from the humor. At the same time, a control movie (a weather information show— very boring for most people) was shown for two weeks to the same two groups of elderly patients, with and without the skin condition. Neither group had a decrease in skin water loss or increase in testosterone. These results do make sense because stress has been shown to decrease testosterone levels and increase water loss from skin.

Of course, the notion that "laughter is the best medicine" has been around since Norman Cousins, M.D. popularized it decades ago in his book <u>Anatomy of an Illness</u> that describes his use of Marx brothers' movies to cure himself of a serious disease. We could all use more humor in our lives; it is not frivolous.

Stress Reduction Techniques

Dr. James Oschman is an expert in the field of energy medicine. I first met him in 2003 when I started my training in Frequency Specific Microcurrent (FSM), a form of energy medicine with which I have experienced great success in my practice. I have used FSM for stress reduction, post traumatic stress disorder (PTSD), concussion, and other brain disorders, as well as many other medical conditions. I have also incorporated FSM into facial rejuvenation, an extraordinary approach to non-surgical face and skin enhancement.

One of the great surprises that I have learned about health over the years is that we are energy beings. Our bodies operate on energy.

There are frequencies that each organ system and tissue operate on that, when disturbed, cause dysfunction. This is the why and how Frequency Specific Microcurrent is able to access the body and work so quickly to heal. FSM is the secret weapon of my practice-just ask my patients. For a video discussion of why I love FSM go here:

https://dr-anne-marie-
fine.mykajabi.com/p/frequencyspecificmicrocurrent

Dr. Oschman describes the body as a living matrix (of which collagen is a primary component) and semi-conductor; the entire living matrix is simultaneously a mechanical, vibrational, energetic, electric, and informational network. Albert Szent-Gyorgyi, a Nobel Prize winner, states, "Life is too rapid and subtle to be explained by slow-moving chemical reactions and nerve impulses." Viewing the body as an electrical being living on an electrical planet completely responsive to the earth's electromagnetic field provides a new framework for understanding how the body really works.

Let's use the heart as an example. Its very health is measured by an electrocardiogram. In fact, the heart generates the largest electromagnetic field in the body. The electric field of the heart, as measured in an electrocardiogram (ECG), is about 60 times greater than the brain waves recorded in an electroencephalogram (EEG), and extends several feet out from the body. The brain also has its own electric field. Let's see how connecting to another electrical grid, the earth, could affect our own electrical milieu and stress levels.

Earthing

Many experts have rediscovered the benefits of walking barefoot on the earth and connecting to the earth's electromagnetic grid. This is called earthing or grounding. The earth functions as a free reservoir of electrons, with these electrons freely taken up into the body from the feet; it is well established that electrons neutralize free radicals. In fact, electrons function as potent antioxidants.

Throughout most of history, people have walked either barefoot or clad in animal skin footwear. They slept on the ground or on animal skins. Thus, the earth's abundant supply of electrons was freely able to enter the body nearly constantly. The body, an electrical conduit or semi-conductor, used them to create a stable bioelectric environment necessary for proper function of all body systems. This is how humans evolved. Today, we are completely cut off from this endless supply of electrons as we wear shoes that are not conductive, since they are usually made of rubber or rubber-soled, and we no longer sleep on the ground. Come to think of it, this may be why camping out in the wilderness on the ground is so refreshing, even accounting for the fact that the ground is very hard and you may not sleep as well from a comfort point of view. And free electrons, remember, are very potent antioxidants. These antioxidants are responsible for the clinical observations from grounding experiments such as:

- Beneficial changes in heart rate
- Decreased levels of inflammation
- Decreased blood viscosity

The decrease in levels of inflammation is a big benefit, as inflammation has been found to promote many chronic diseases of aging including wrinkle formation. Any food, supplement, or mind-body technique that can decrease inflammation is absolutely critical in maintaining one's health and preventing premature aging, including preventing wrinkles on the face.

In fact, earthing can be considered an anti-aging strategy for the same reasons—chronic inflammation is driving the aging process all over the body. One of the leading theories of aging is the free-radical theory, which states that free radicals cause a cascade of molecules losing and gaining electrons that leads to an accumulation of damage to the body, including inflammation, which is what aging is all about.

In one small study, earthing was also shown to objectively decrease cortisol, our stress hormone, and subjectively decrease pain and stress. In this study, patients who complained of sleep disturbances, stress (anxiety, depression, and irritability), and pain were instructed to sleep grounded on conductive mattresses. All but one participant reported falling asleep more quickly, and all reported fewer nighttime awakenings. Daytime energy levels were restored and cortisol rhythms normalized.

Maybe Clark ought to sleep outside on the grass, Ha! (•‿•)

In another double-blind study, earthing was shown to affect the autonomic nervous system by moving participants out of sympathetic nervous system activation (fight or flight) to parasympathetic (relaxing) mode. This is the direction we want to move in for our stress reduction techniques—into parasympathetic tone. I am finding that many people have become "stuck" in the sympathetic nervous system mode and this is why they have so much trouble relaxing.

The beautiful thing about earthing is that it is free and can be done anywhere. All you need to do is take off your shoes and contact the earth in bare feet. Sometimes all it takes is 20 minutes to notice a reduction in pain. There is, however, another consideration and that is that the place in which you earth does make a difference. The presence of water nearby, in particular the ocean, enhances the effects of earthing since water is such an effective conductor. So walking barefoot on the beach is the best place to earth.

I have earthed on beaches from Newport and Laguna Beach to Monte Carlo, Barcelona, Hawaii, Vancouver, the Italian Riviera, and the truly wild and windswept beaches of enchanting Ireland. In fact, whenever I travel, I try to find a beach within hours of landing to earth on, as it reduces the effects of jet lag and really grounds me after travel that traverses several time zones. It is part of my jet-lag protocol, which also includes FSM programmed for jet lag, which I run on the flight while actually traveling through different time zones. These two amazing secrets are how I am able to travel around the world with virtually no jet lag, and hit the ground running as soon as I land. Not having to deal with jet lag is an absolute treasure.

The next best place to earth is on grass that still has some dew on it in the morning. In some European countries, walking barefoot in the morning on the dew-covered grass is a time-honored tradition and still practiced by many people.

By connecting to the earth, you can access a completely free source of antioxidants that can help heal injuries, reduce inflammation and stress, and prevent free-radical damage. For most people, this is something that is readily accessible. There is a reason why going barefoot makes you feel so good!! This has been known forever. Even Adam and Eve were barefoot in the garden. Come to think of it, maybe this is why people who garden feel so good—they are connected to the earth.

Beauty Boost

Earthing

- Anti-inflammatory
- Anti-aging
- Free source of antioxidants
- Relaxing
- Reduces pain

Spending Time in Nature (with your shoes on)

At no other time in history have we been so disconnected to nature. As humans became more urban and more cocooned in their cars and energy-efficient homes (which render them airtight), the values of nature and just being outdoors, suffered a regrettable decline. We are paying the price of this disconnect with our bodies; the decline of time spent in nature corresponds to the increase in stress, anxiety, frustration, and physical ailments.

Spending time in nature has begun to generate some interesting research documenting that even just looking out of a window at nature can be beneficial to human health and wellbeing. Specifically, contact with nature has been reported to reduce stress, improve attention (even in ADHD children), increase longevity, reduce blood pressure, and improve mood. However, the great outdoors is having a hard time competing with our electronic gadgets and social media bids for attention. Visits to our beautiful National Parks have reported a decline over the last 20 years.

The stress-relieving aspect of nature therapy may be the key element here. Who hasn't found a day at the beach, hiking, or walking through a forest completely relaxing and rejuvenating? This has been known for many years, and city planners have this idea in mind when they plan for city parks. Central Park is but one example of this natural oasis in the middle of dense urbanity.

The Japanese have been studying the positive health effect of spending time in a forest through research. They even have a name for it: Forest Bathing, or Shinrin-yoku. Apparently, this phenomenon is so well known that they have nature therapy sites that are located in a forest where the prescription is "take two hours of forest bathing and call me in the morning."

In one field study that was conducted over 24 different forests in Japan, some truly remarkable effects were discovered. Participants were instructed to walk through a forest for about 15 minutes and then to just view the forest for about 15 minutes on one day, followed the next day by walking in and viewing a city for the same amount of time. During the forest bathing times, their pulse rates, cortisol levels, blood pressure, and heart-rate variability were lower. At the same time, their stress response favored the opposite reaction of fight or flight—relaxation—as compared to their time walking in and viewing a city. That is not a lot of time in which to produce such impressive results in stress reduction! Even more amazing is an earlier study that demonstrated a reduction in glycation, that sugar-induced wrinkling process, by walking in forest air. Who knew that walking in a forest can be a beauty boost?

More recent research has been performed with forest bathing that quantifies some of these benefits. Specifically, after merely sitting in the forest, the subjects showed a 12.4% decrease in cortisol levels, a 7% decrease in stress, a 5.8% decrease in heart rate, and a 55% increase in relaxation as measured by the parasympathetic activity (the opposite of our fight or flight system). The control group was again subjected to an urban environment.

In another study of forest bathing in both men and women, immune function was increased by nearly 40% and lasted 30 days following a 3-day, 2-night trip to the forest. This was due to the effects of phytoncides, or wood essential oils, which waft out of trees and permeate the forest air.

Just sitting in nature is turning out to be preventive medicine at its best. Even looking outside of your window at greenery has been shown to reduce the stress response and adding plants to your environment is helpful as well. I recommend getting outside for a walk every day, even if you don't have a nearby forest to visit. Just getting some fresh air is beneficial. *Like looking out my backyard is relaxing*

Hildegard von Bingen, a twelfth-century Christian mystic, composer, poet, writer, the first known woman physician, and abbess, was way ahead of her time in many aspects of life including the value of nature. Called the Sybil of the Rhine, she was blessed with Divine revelation. She had an unusual creation-based cosmology that centered on nature. Indeed, Hildegard was in love with nature, even coining a word "verititas" which means the greening and healing power of nature. Even this Medieval Renaissance woman believed that spending time in nature was healing, 800 years before the resurgence of interest in nature as medicine.

Hildegard was a visionary in all things ecological and believed we humans were tasked with protecting the earth as we cannot live without it. She went on to write extensive compendiums on healing utilizing the natural world and plants, and some consider her to be the Mother of Naturopathic Medicine. How prescient of her to recognize the natural world as a gift so fundamental to our human survival.

Tai Chi

Tai chi, a form of Chinese martial arts and considered in the United States to be a low-impact mind-body exercise, has been practiced for millennia for health, fitness, and wellbeing in the East and continues to gain popularity in the West. Tai chi has been proven to decrease anxiety and depression. Tai chi requires no equipment whatsoever, not even any special clothes. It is typically performed outdoors in a park. If you perform it barefoot and outdoors on grass, you will get the added benefit of earthing. Tai chi is very gentle on the body, decreases stress, and promotes the cultivation of chi, or energy, in the body.

As mentioned previously, we are energy beings. We have a very prominent physical body, it is the part of us that gets the most attention; but energy is what animates us and makes all our parts work. The free flow of energy in our bodies is what keeps us healthy. In traditional Chinese medicine, to name one philosophy of medicine that focuses on energy in our body, diagnoses are given based on where the energy flow is "blocked" in the body. The insertion of acupuncture needles in certain points along a meridian is employed to release the blockage and restore free flow of energy along a meridian that usually involves one organ. Tai chi is beneficial because it not only works on a physical level to increase range of motion with joints and decrease stress and anxiety, it also promotes free flow of energy.

In addition, tai chi also fights free radicals, those destructive forces of aging. In one recent study of postmenopausal women, in a randomized, placebo-controlled, clinical study that lasted only six months, it was found that green tea reduced a marker of oxidative stress (which reflects free-radical damage) by 40%—a nice figure. Tai chi was found to decrease the same marker by 60%—even better! But the synergistic effect of the group who consumed green tea AND performed tai chi one hour three times a week, reduced this marker by a whopping 73%.

While I was writing this book, I happened to speak to a friend about Tai chi and aging and she provided me with a beautiful illustration of how it benefits skin and the aging process. A few years ago, a new client came to see my friend, a woman who appeared to be in her sixties. Imagine my friend's surprise when the woman turned out to be 94! My friend asked her what her secret was and discovered that the woman had started a new business in her sixties: teaching pregnant women Tai chi. My friend last saw this woman when she was 104, still radiant and radiating life purpose, independent, and glowing with health and vitality. Now that's the kind of older woman we should be emulating.

The anti-aging effects of Tai chi may also have something to do with glycation levels, as one study showed that, after 12 months, glycation levels *and* markers of oxidative stress (both promoters of skin wrinkling) decreased in Tai chi participants.

In a pilot study of 273 experienced practitioners of Tai chi compared to 263 age- and ethnicity-matched controls, it was found that Tai chi had favorable epigenetic effects on the methylation of the six gene regions examined, notably slowing the age-related trends for DNA methylation losses or gains. A fun fact is that the gene region that showed the greatest improvement was that of a gene controlling

DNA double-strand break repair. Being able to repair DNA strand breaks is extraordinarily useful as we age! Although this is a preliminary study of just a few gene regions, I found it interesting that *all* six showed favorable changes.

The authors of this study were trying to see *why* Tai chi studies support a positive effect on many different conditions, such as balance control, flexibility, cardiovascular fitness (in the absence of it being aerobic activity), falls in the elderly, osteoarthritis, rheumatoid arthritis, hypertension, bone mineral density, neuromuscular function, respiratory, immune, and hormone function. Also positively supported are psychological responses including depression and quality of life issues like pain management, sleep quality, and stress reduction; the subject of this chapter.

Tai chi is becoming better known as an epigenetic modifier of immune health as well. Recent information has come to light that Tai chi actually modulates the genes responsible for inflammation, which, in turn, regulates the immune system. What else does inflammation promote? Skin aging, wrinkling, and loss of elasticity. These kinds of studies highlight the promise that Tai chi and other mind-body therapies have in turning off the pro-inflammatory, and hence pro-disease and *pro-aging*, genes in the body. This is revolutionary information, and one more way to **turn *on* your beauty genes.**

I am a regular practitioner of Tai chi and I love it. It is something that you can fit into your life easily because, once you learn it, you can do it at home or in a park at your leisure. You don't have to change into special clothes or fit into someone else's schedule.

Yoga is another moving meditation that has been linked with healthier aging. It is a time-honored way to reduce cortisol, reduce depression, improve sleep, and restore vitality. All of these measures are beneficial for aging of not only the face, but the whole body system, joints, muscles, and ligaments. Flexibility declines with age, and contributes to feeling old. After all, when you can't get around as easily, it is quite common to just blame it on getting older. If you have ever seen pictures or know any lifelong yoga practitioners, you would have to conclude that it is youth-promoting in mind, body, and spirit.

Meditation and Deep Breathing

Meditation in all its forms largely involves sitting still, emptying the mind, and focusing on your breathing or a specific phrase or mantra. It is cultivating stillness and inner focus. In the West, meditation is used to reduce stress, anxiety, blood pressure, and calm the body, while also benefiting cognitive abilities and positive emotional regulation. Many studies support its use in reducing the stress hormone, cortisol, in people.

Transcendental Meditation

The most studies performed on meditation involve a form called Transcendental Meditation (TM). TM is a meditation practice that one does for 20 minutes twice daily using a mantra. Researchers have been studying TM for over 40 years and have amassed quite a body of evidence for the results TM can provide for its practitioners.

Peer-reviewed published research on the TM technique has found a wide range of health benefits including:

- Greater inner calm throughout the day
- Reduced cortisol
- Normalized blood pressure
- Reduced insomnia
- Lower risk of heart attack and stroke
- Reduced anxiety and depression
- Improved brain function and memory

Mindfulness Meditation

In the spirit of this book, how to epigenetically turn on and off specific genes relating to aging, mindfulness meditation has now been studied and found to actually turn down the genes for inflammation and, since inflammation is intimately connected to facial aging, we have a basis to connect the dots and conclude that meditation is good for healthy aging and, specifically, can reduce facial wrinkling.

The best definition of mindfulness comes from the founder of Mindfulness-Based Stress Reduction (MBSR) and author of Full Catastrophe Living, Jon Kabat-Zinn. He defines it as "paying attention on purpose, in the present moment, and nonjudgmentally, to the unfolding of experience moment to moment." Another way to put it is to simply be present in the now with whatever you are doing, while really paying attention.

There have now been many randomized, controlled trials of mindfulness-based therapies and what they conclude is that MBSR can reduce chronic pain and anxiety, reduce stress, and improve quality of life in healthy volunteers and also cancer survivors.

Let's use dishwashing as an example. Don't tell anyone, but I actually like to do dishes and believe the only use for an automatic dishwasher is as a drying rack. That means I do a lot of dishes. But did you know you can use dishwashing as an exercise in mindfulness?

Here's what that looks like. When you are washing dishes, pay attention to the scent of the dish soap you use (I like lavender-scented), the temperature of the water (the warm water feels so good on a cold day), and the froth of the suds. Think of it as a bubble bath for your hands. Really immerse yourself in the scrubbing, washing, and rinsing of your dishes. Place them carefully and mindfully in your drying rack. Thoughts will occur to you, but place your attention more on your breath and the task in front of you. I find this to be very stress relieving and the complete opposite of most of the rest of my days, which may involve multitasking, interruptions, and stealth stress bombs detonating randomly in my day.

So imagine my surprise when I read about a study in 2015 where student and faculty researchers at Florida State University found that mindfully washing dishes calms the mind and decreases stress by 27%. I knew I was on to something! And I like the idea that mindfulness meditation does not have to be a formal practice that involves special accoutrements, but can be done quite casually during the day. Just be present with what you are doing in the moment.

A recent study examined a group of people experienced in mindfulness meditation and a control group of people with no meditation experience for one eight-hour period. The experienced meditators were asked to meditate for the eight hours, so this was an intensive day of mindfulness meditation, and the control group was asked to enjoy leisure activities in the same setting for the same amount of time. Now here's where it gets interesting. After the eight-hour intervention period, the meditators had *favorable epigenetic changes* to their stress response and the participants who simply enjoyed leisure activities (which also are believed to be good for stress; after all, these people were not working or performing math problems) did not show changes to the epigenetic markers that were studied. These changes included changes in the genes' coding for inflammation, lowering them. We know inflammation drives aging and facial wrinkling, so this suggests we have another strategy to employ to not only help us find our center and enjoy more peaceful days and nights, but to age more gently.

Harvard researchers performed an eight-week study of mindfulness meditation that attempted to go past the already reported benefits of peacefulness and physical stress reduction, into actual brain changes. What they found has profound implication for our brain health and for our ability to change our brains.

The participants logged, on average, 27 minutes per day of mindfulness meditation. The analysis of magnetic resonance images taken of the brain before and after the intervention found increased gray-matter density in the hippocampus, the memory center, and in structures associated with self-awareness, compassion, and introspection. Participant-reported reductions in stress also were correlated with decreased gray-matter density in the amygdala, the seat of anxiety and stress. The study illustrated that our brains are "plastic" and can change, and did change in this eight-week study of mindfulness meditation.

Loving-Kindness Meditation

Another kind of meditation that has recently garnered more attention through its research-based findings is Loving-Kindness Meditation (LKM), a meditation with roots in Buddhism. In this meditation, the emotions of love and compassion are actively aroused and directed towards self and others. I first learned LKM about 20 years ago, when it appeared to be a rather obscure form of meditation; but its devotees are growing.

Essentially in this meditation, one is directed to love everyone, the "Golden Rule," the absolute top commandment given by Jesus, and found in nearly all established religions. And yet, not only do most people not love their enemy, they don't even love themselves. This simple-sounding tenet is at the heart of our humanity as spiritual beings.

Pierre Teilhard de Chardin SJ, priest and paleontologist (an unusual combination, to say the least), had the following to say about love:

> "The day will come when, after harnessing space, the winds, the tides, gravitation, we shall harness for God the energies of love. And, on that day, for the second time in the history of the world, humanity will have discovered fire."
>
> (Fire of Love : Encountering the Holy Spirit (2006) by Donald Goergen, p. 92)

> "Love is the most universal, the most tremendous and the most mystical of cosmic forces. Love is the primal and universal psychic energy. Love is a sacred reserve of energy; it is like the blood of spiritual evolution."
>
> (The Spirit of the Earth, 1931, VI, 32, 33, 34)

Research has found that Loving-Kindness meditation generates greater self-compassion, which is linked to lower levels of anxiety and depression, increases brain volume in the areas that regulate emotions (meditation grows your brain), contributes to social connectedness, and, as a bonus, acts like an internal youth promoter by increasing telomere length, a biological marker of aging. This is truly astonishing: that our minds actually exert control over aging.

LKM and other forms of meditation are proven to decrease cortisol, your stress hormone, which will lower your stress-induced accelerated aging, help you get your beauty sleep, and increase telomere length, a marker of aging. Meditation is one of the most powerful beauty boosters because it is free, can be taken anywhere and done anytime, and it provides a multitude of benefits on the mind and body.

How do you perform LKM? This meditation can be adapted to your own particular needs, but here is a beginner script that can get you started. The entire meditation should take no more than 15 minutes.

Loving-Kindness Meditation

Sit comfortably, with your spine straight and your hands held loosely in your lap, or in traditional meditation position, palms up on your knees. Close your eyes for this exercise. Take a deep breath and let it out. No need to count, just make sure you can feel your belly expanding on the inhale. Take a few deep breaths, from your heart center, and allow yourself to settle into this exercise.

Step 1

Stay in this step for the first week or so until you can feel the love vibrating in your entire being. There is no point in progressing on to loving others until you can love yourself.

This part of the meditation is focused on you. The purpose is to ground you in a foundation of self-love, without which it is impossible to truly love and care for another. While you are breathing deeply, imagine someone who loves you deeply (a parent, mentor, lover, friend) standing on your right side. As you move through the statements below, start adding other people who love you unabashedly until you have a circle of loved ones sending you love and goodwill. Bask in this love and really receive it while you say, or even sing, the following out loud, in your head (three times):

May I be safe

May I be healthy

May I be happy

May I live with ease

Step 2

Now repeat the phrases for someone for whom you have unconditional love. It can be the person who you are imagining on your right or someone else who easily evokes this unconditional love. Repeat these phrases:

May he/she be safe

May he/she be healthy

May he/she be happy

May he/she live with ease

Step 3

On this next round, choose a neutral person, such as the checkout clerk at the grocery store or the postman. You neither like nor dislike this person. Repeat the phrases, which you let reverberate through your entire body, mind, heart, and soul, and physically feel it as you send it out to the recipients:

May he/she be safe

May he/she be healthy

May he/she be happy

May he/she live with ease

Step 4

This time you will choose a difficult person for you, someone who has hurt you, or who you resent. This may be more difficult for you, but the idea is that the warmth and goodwill your meditation has been bathing you in, allows you to send out love and kindness to this difficult person. If you cannot stay in your loving space, you can precede the phrases with the qualifier "To the best of my ability I wish that you be...." If you simply cannot feel love towards this person, simply go back to Step 2, your benefactor to regenerate your vibration of love.

May he/she be safe

May he/she be healthy

May he/she be happy

May he/she live with ease

Step 5

In this iteration, you will be sending out loving-kindness to everybody in the world, evoking a feeling of oneness and its resulting peace, compassion, and empathy for even strangers in this world.

May all be safe

May all be healthy

May all be happy

May all live with ease

If you have made this meditation part of your daily practice, you can now expand your abilities by trying it outside in the real world in situations that are fraught with conflict. You can try this at work when you get into a confrontation with a boss or coworker, or are simply nervous before a presentation. You can try this when a difficult conversation comes up with your loved ones. In these instances, you will keep your eyes open, stay present, but simply drop into your heart and repeat the phrases above while actively sending love and kindness out to the person standing in front of you.

Not all stress reduction techniques are the same, nor will they work for everybody. We are all unique individuals and must try a few to find something that works for us. But I believe stress reduction is important for everybody; in particular for those who seem to have a hard time finding one that works.

While many extoll the virtues of meditation, some people find that they simply cannot turn off their minds and reap the full benefits of this technique. In this case, beginning with a simple breathing meditation is the way to go. Deep breathing alone has been found to decrease cortisol and blood pressure. In fact, you can try this yourself the next time you have an opportunity to have your blood pressure taken. After it is taken for the first time, pause, and for about two minutes slow down your breathing and take deeper breaths. Then retake your blood pressure. It is bound to be lower.

Back in the 1970s, Herbert Benson, MD, a researcher at Harvard University Medical School, coined the term "the relaxation response" after conducting research on people who practiced transcendental meditation. The relaxation response, in Benson's words, is "an opposite, involuntary response that causes a reduction in the activity of the sympathetic nervous system." This causes an increase in the opposite: the parasympathetic nervous system, the relaxed and calm state. Achieving the parasympathetic state is the goal of stress reduction techniques.

Since then, studies on the relaxation response have documented the following short-term benefits to the nervous system:

- Lower blood pressure
- Improved blood circulation
- Lower heart rate
- Slower respiratory rate
- Less anxiety
- Lower blood cortisol levels
- Less stress
- Deeper relaxation

There are many methods to elicit the relaxation response, including, progressive muscle relaxation, different forms of energy healing, acupuncture, massage, breathing techniques, prayer, meditation, Tai chi, and yoga. This response can also be achieved by choosing a word, sound, phrase, prayer, or by focusing on your breathing. It doesn't have to be very complicated and, if you are just beginning, make it easy on yourself.

A simple meditation for beginners would look like this:

- Sit or lie in a comfortable position
- Close your eyes
- Breathe normally, but focus on your breathing
- Observe thoughts that come up, but let them pass without judgement

There are many variations on this simple meditation involving more complex breath work (such as counting to 4 on the inhale, holding for 4, and counting to another 4 on the exhale), focusing on certain words or phrases, or looking into a candle flame. Meditation can be done for 2-3 minutes at a time at the beginning. With practice and dedication, a longer meditation practice can be achieved.

Recently I found the holy grail of guided meditations combined with brain state technology, conveniently packaged on an iPod-like device. I call it the IAMFINE® Beauty Sleep System and have it available on my website www.drannemariefine.com. This device combines a listening experience with binaural beats with special LED glasses that emit flashing blue lights designed to help change brain waves into a more relaxed and receptive state. This device comes preloaded with several guided meditations on stress reduction, beauty, and sleep, and has the ability to have additional programs loaded on to it from an extensive library of programs that deal with issues such as weight loss, business success, personal growth, coping with cancer, and more.

To use this device you simply lie or sit down, put the ear buds in and the glasses on, and select the guided meditation program that you wish to listen to, press a button, and voila; you will calm yourself down and enjoy all the benefits of meditation in about 20 minutes. I now use it every day—it is my go-to meditation device. And while I have long been a fan of binaural-beat technology embedded in other brainwave entrainment programs that increase relaxation, change production of hormones, and decrease anxiety and stress, this is the first program I have found that incorporates the flashing LED lights, which have their own effects on brainwave entrainment.

The internet abounds with resources on all kinds of meditation including guided meditations and downloads. Browse the internet and see what appeals to you. There are also many apps available on your smart phones that can get you started on the way to greater peace and relaxation. Meditation has gone mainstream and can now be accessed easily through technology. These days, there is no excuse or barrier to meditation, or mindfulness-based training. Just find the time to do it.

Prayer

Prayer and regular church attendance have been shown to decrease stress, improve health and even longevity. Having a strong connection to Spirit is essential to living a life that is guided. How many of us have had strong experiences of being guided to doing something that we would have not normally done, that led to a complete change in our life or our life's mission?

When you live a life that aligns your soul with Spirit, you are allowing for guidance to work in your life, and allowing for your life to flow. If you continually resist this inner "call to action" this is where exhaustion, stress, and ill health find a home in your heart.

One way to think of this is to imagine that your life's journey is a river, flowing in one direction. If you allow the river to hold you and support you, your trip downstream goes along much more smoothly. If you are constantly trying to swim upstream, your journey becomes very exhausting and can lead to resentment and bitterness about how hard your life is.

I am reminded of a plaque that a friend of mine has on her desk, which reads:

"If you want to make God laugh, tell Him your plans."

As for praying, it too is a form of meditation, an opening up and request to the Divine for intervention, a time for silence and introspection, a time to receive grace. Focusing on the Mystery of

Life, on faith, on our intimate connection to the Divine can foster serenity and peacefulness.

Cultural Expectations and Aging

Much of aging, it turns out, is culturally inspired. People seem to buy into the common cultural myths of what getting old means. They seem to collectively understand that poorer health and disability is simply a function of time. That everyone slows down when they get older, and multiple prescription drugs are necessary in order to function at all.

Menopause is one phase of life that represents this cultural conditioning. In the United States, menopause is a dreaded time of life that represents loss of beauty, sexual attraction, vitality, and has horrific side effects like hot flashes, insomnia, mood swings, weight gain—weight gain is *huge*. We even have a name for it: Menopause Belly. Nobody wants to go through menopause, let alone explore what is on the other side. It's really all downhill from there, is the thought.

I remember once in my practice I had a new patient from the Middle East. Her interpreter arrived a little bit before her, and so the interpreter asked me a simple question. What kinds of patients do you see? I told her I saw a variety of patients, but that most of my practice involved women and menopause, autoimmune disease, digestive issues, and the interpreter immediately looked baffled. I asked her what was wrong and she wanted to know why the menopausal women needed to see me, a doctor. I said, "For the hot flashes, anxiety, insomnia, and other symptoms of menopause." She was very surprised and offered that in the Middle East, women did not suffer from these symptoms of menopause, that it was considered a very natural passage through which every woman passed without incident.

She further explained that when women in the Middle East give birth, they go to bed for a few months and their mothers and sisters come into her and her husband's home to take care of her, the baby and any other children, and the husband in terms of meals, housework, and the like. In this way, the new mothers were given ample time for their bodies to heal and their strength to come back from the task of being pregnant and giving birth. Contrast this to our policy of women working right up to the due date and getting back to the office in six weeks! Does pampering the new mom's reproductive organs make for an easier menopausal transition? Or is it a different cultural expectation?

And then you have the other side of the equation: the people who refuse to age, who refuse to buy into the aging myths which literally are aging us! The baby boomers are famous for this. An entire generation of people born between 1945 and 1964 have thrown out their parents' cultural expectations of the aging process and, as a result are living longer, working longer, and being active and productive well into their elderly years. I can see how my parents' generation looked old in their fifties, and slowed down and waited for death and disability to claim them.

Well, I was fortunate to have a mother who defied these cultural expectations and not only had a brilliant career as a nurse and therapist, but worked into her 70s. At the same time that woman could out dance any person on the dance floor and could put any wedding attendee, including the bride and groom, to shame with her excellent dancing skills, honed over decades. We are not talking about the waltz here, but the Lindy, East Coast Swing, and her favorite, the Jitterbug. She was unbelievable.

One of the most fun weddings I ever attended was with my mother a few years ago when she, my daughter, and I, all avid dancers, stormed the dance floor and danced our hearts out with each other. The irony was, my mom had Stage 4 terminal cancer at that point, but was determined that it was not going to interfere with her fun and dancing at that most joyous of occasions, the wedding. It is mind over matter. You make your own way in this world, and create your own world with your mind, your attitudes, your beliefs, and your thoughts. It simply would not have occurred to my mom that she should sit out this dance, or wedding, simply because she had a terminal illness. Especially if she had to miss an opportunity to dance!

My mother is a prime example that aging does not have to diminish your energy and enjoyment of hobbies- in fact zest for life makes you beautiful.

A Connection to Spirit

A connection to Spirit is also essential to joyful, healthy living. An understanding of our Divine nature and connection to God facilitates the unfolding of our soul essence, and fulfills our purpose here on earth. Each one of us comes here with unique and powerful gifts that were given to us to use on our journey through our earthly life. Our individual gifts, personalities, and physical forms provide astonishing diversity to humankind. It is absolutely crazy that we seek to be just like other people, look like them, and act like them when our own gifts and look are equally compelling. We aspire to conformity for reasons that include acceptance, peer pressure, societal pressures, and religious doctrinal pressure, when really we all come from the same source, are made from the same material, and are here to dazzle and interact with each other in all of our infinite glory.

Let's all just be ourselves. It's less demanding than trying to be someone else. And authenticity is magnetic and youthful!

There is no woman on earth as beautiful as the woman who has discerned her soul's purpose and has embraced it. This woman radiates gratitude and love within whatever capacity she moves. Some women were called to be mothers and have poured their life's energy into the nurturing and caring for their families. Some women have been called to be healers, public servants, lawyers, accountants, bankers, entrepreneurs, bent on making the world a better place with their innovative products or services. Many women do more than one at the same time or in sequence. Some women are called to protect Mother Earth and other women are called to explore the cosmos. Everyone comes here with gifts and they are not all the same. Everyone is here to shine their special light. Do not hide your light under a bushel!

One of the problems with aging is that some women seem to forget their purpose. Once the children are grown and launched, retirement is achieved from the workforce, some women don't know what to do with themselves. This in itself is very aging. In her book titled The Gift of Years: Growing Older Gracefully, Joan Chittister expresses it this way:

"The world has been upside down for so long, it is almost impossible to believe anymore that the meaning of life is not about *doing*. The notion that it is about *being*—being caring, being interested, being honest, being truthful, being available, being spiritual, being involved with the important things of life, of living—is so rare, so unspoken of, as to be obtuse. We don't even know what meaning means anymore."

Indeed, it is important to remember that we are human *beings*, not human doings.

In another book, The Grace in Dying by Kathleen Dowling Singh (which my mother bequeathed me) the author explains the process of our lives in this way. In essence, we go through life with very heavy body armor, vigorously defending our ego from the world based on the trauma and life experiences we have gone though as younger people, propping up our personalities and the persona we wish to project to the world. This is exhausting, and uses up precious energy that could be used for healing and growth. The grace in dying, and the gift, is when we can finally discard all our masks and become the person we were meant to be all along, and integrate with our spirit. In the words of the author, "It is a movement from personality, to soul, to Spirit."

And if we can do it well before our dying, integrating with our true spirit imbues us with the energy and light and will to live and live well, contributing our time and talents in whichever way is appropriate for us, well into our later years. And I feel that this is THE rare and true secret of aging well. We must have passion and purpose for living and being here now. There is no time like the present for embracing this gift of life. Be alive!

Beauty Boost

- Find your bliss and follow it
- Don't wait until you are dying to live
- Be authentic
- Express yourself and live a congruent life
- Don't worry what other people think of you...it's none of your business

To find beauty in everyone you must see beauty in everyone, then announce that you see it, for in announcing it, you place it there in their reality.

Do not miss a single chance—not one single opportunity—to tell someone how wonderful they are, how special they are, how important to you they are, how incredible as a person they are, how beautiful they are inside and out. Do not miss a single opening in which to insert such a comment, genuinely felt and genuinely meant.

Make it your life's mission today to bring to the attention of another just how extraordinary they are. Say it. Say it. SAY it. Their heart is waiting to know that their own best thought about themselves can be believed.

Neale Donald Walsch

Applying the information

The Minimalist

- Meditate. Find a simple meditation practice that works for you and start with only 5 minutes once daily. Work up to 10 minutes.
- Try earthing when you have the opportunity.

The Middle Way: Accompanying the above,

- Switch to The Loving Kindness Meditation (about 15 minutes) or another meditation that is guided and lasts longer. Use your internet or smart phone to find one that works for you.
- Review your beliefs about aging objectively and replace limiting beliefs with empowering beliefs.

The Beauty Buff: In Addition to All of the above,

- Add yoga or Tai chi to bring more movement and energy.

CHAPTER EIGHT

Sleeping for Beauty

*"They don't call it Beauty Sleep for nothing! Sleep is the ultimate cosmetic!—**Dr.Fine***

Beauty Sleep

SLEEP IS ESSENTIAL to emotional and physical health. Inadequate sleep over a period of time increases the risks for obesity, diabetes, heart disease, and depression. It will also sap your face of vitality, radiance, and youth! Everyone has experienced the dull skin, under-eye darkness and circles, and generally haggard appearance after a bad night of sleep, or an all-nighter. However, in these stressful times, chronic sleep deprivation is more the norm than the exception, with obvious implications for our skin-aging process. There is a reason why it is called Beauty Sleep.

While the Fountain of Youth has been searched for endlessly, instead of an elixir, beauty serum, or cream, what if we could simply sleep our way to radiant skin? Sleep is the ultimate cosmetic! And it is free. What is it about sleep that fuels skin vitality? And how can we ditch our modern sleep disruptors and get more time between the sheets?

Sleep is the time that your skin rejuvenates and repairs daily damage. Deep sleep may be called beauty sleep because the production of human growth hormone surges during sleep and contributes to robust collagen formation in the skin. Growth hormone also helps repair and rebuild other body tissues like muscle and bone. Sleep is also a time for the production of other proteins that repair damaged cells and grow new cells while performing certain housecleaning functions, like taking out the cellular garbage.

Sleep deprivation, on the other hand, slows down the normal wound healing properties of skin and destroys your collagen. This is also true with stress. Chronic stress, with its accompanying high levels of cortisol, can interfere with sleep. Cortisol, as you know, increases inflammation resulting in breakdown of collagen, so it makes sense that a study in the *Journal of Investigative Dermatology* (2001) demonstrated that women who are sleep-deprived had dysfunctional skin-barrier function, which promoted increased trans-epidermal water loss and much higher levels of inflammatory chemicals in their blood. When you have high levels of water evaporating out of your skin it leads to dehydrated skin that shows all the wrinkles, particularly the fine lines, because moisture in the skin plumps up the skin. This is the same scenario observed in women experiencing chronic stress or anxiety or depression. Insomnia, stress, anxiety, and depression are all instrumental in ruining our complexions.

Moreover, a 2010 study in the British Medical Journal found that people who had a full night of sleep (eight-plus hours) versus the sleep-deprived (31 hours of wakefulness after a night of reduced sleep) were rated as more attractive and healthy. Lack of sleep can make us more unattractive rather quickly. In a similar study of people with obstructive sleep apnea, the ones who used a positive-airway-pressure device at night, and thus slept better, were rated as being more attractive and younger looking. An unexpected observation was that their forehead wrinkles were reduced. Quick! Dive for the covers and stay there!

Furthermore, a recent study demonstrated that a **single** night of partial sleep deprivation activated a gene-expression pattern consistent with biological aging. This proves a causal link of sleep deprivation to the molecular processes associated with aging. This is why sleep is such an important epigenetic factor for health and beauty.

The evidence shows that, for many people today, getting their beauty sleep is just not happening. Prescriptions for sleeping pills and over-the-counter sleep aids continue to rise as people turn to help for trying to get some sleep, which is something that should be free…and easy. From 1999-2010, there was a 29% increase in "sleep disturbance" as the reason given for an office visit to a doctor. So, it is probably not surprising that, from 2006-2011, the market for over-the-counter sleep aids grew 31% with the biggest growth category being natural and homeopathic products.

The National Sleep Foundation currently recommends 7-8 hours of sleep per night for adults. According to a Gallup poll from 2013, only 59% of Americans reach that goal, while 40% get fewer than 7 hours. The average hours slept per night in 2013 were 6.8. Contrast that to 1942, when the average hours slept per night were 7.9. The number of hours spent sleeping have declined over the last 70 years.

Chronic, long-term sleep disorders affect at least 40 million Americans each year, and an additional 20 million experience the occasional bout of insomnia. Lack of sleep costs an estimated $16 billion in medical costs each year, while the indirect costs and impacts on work, driving, and social activities are much greater. Driving while sleep impaired has been shown to be on par with driving intoxicated. There is no mistaking the fact that millions of people are walking around in a sleep-deprived mode. How many of you have nodded off during a meeting, or at a stop light, or in a movie? Daytime drowsiness is a big problem today and it's not just our looks that are at risk.

Three Culprits That Steal Your Sleep

- Anxiety/Depression/Overactive minds
- Light
- Stimulation

Anxiety/Depression/Overactive Minds

Anxiety, depression, and overactive minds are definite beauty robbers, snatching good sleep out from under you in a sneaky way. We live in an age of anxiety, where to-do lists, deadlines, and responsibilities compete for our attention and time. Anxiety and depression are both associated with sleep problems. Generally, anxious people have a harder time falling asleep, and depressed people usually can fall asleep but find themselves awake at 3:00 am and unable to fall back to sleep. People who can't turn their minds off at night also suffer from an inability to fall, and stay, asleep.

Soothing night time rituals can pave the way for an easier slide into slumberland. One reason it is so hard to wind down at night is that we have so many competing activities to choose from. Our work comes home with us, the chores are never done, the kids/spouse/aging parents need attention, the bills need to be paid, and the sheer variety of mind-numbing entertainment options can keep us up all night if we let them. Never before have so many movies, TV shows, documentaries, news shows, music videos, YouTube blurbs, TED talks, and talk shows been available to us at any time that works for us. When I was growing up, if you missed your favorite TV show's episode for that week, you were simply out of luck.

New studies show that insomnia might be the result of low gamma amino butyric acid (GABA), a neurochemical responsible for decreasing brain activity in many areas that effectively allows the brain to slow down for sleep. In effect, GABA is an inhibitory neurotransmitter whose role it is to turn down the excitatory neurotransmitters in the brain to calm things down. As it turns out, stress depletes the body of GABA, setting up a scenario for concomitant insomnia. Chronic insomniacs were shown to have a 33% lower level of GABA in their brains. Don't worry; there are ways to increase your GABA—through meditation, tai chi, and yoga. There are even GABA supplements.

Interestingly, GABA has a skin connection too. Administering GABA to rats was effective in accelerating wound healing by suppressing inflammation and stimulating new tissue growth. A lack of GABA in the skin is associated with reduced collagen and other structural proteins and poorer barrier function. The connection between stress, sleeping, and skin becomes even clearer. This is one reason that lack of beauty sleep promotes visible signs of aging.

GABA and melatonin, which are discussed under Light Interference a few paragraphs down, are both secreted in the brain. It is significant to note that there is a clear connection between what is going on in the brain and what shows up on our face. The brain-skin connection is something that cannot be avoided in the quest for clear skin and healthy aging.

Power Down

One method to start winding down at night is to "power down" or "unplug" one hour before bedtime. Just like you "power up" your electronics in the morning, at night, one hour before bedtime, "power down" all your electronics and yourself. During this time, it is okay and even preferable to engage in mind-numbing chores such as folding the laundry or finishing up the kitchen chores. But they must be done mindfully which will turn these necessary but unpleasant chores into nighttime moving, mindfulness meditations.

Mindfulness, which was discussed in the previous chapter, is a stress-reduction technique based on focusing your awareness on the current moment. Mindfulness has become very popular in the last few years because it is so effective for anxiety and other stress-related issues, and yet is easily done anytime, anywhere with no needed equipment. It encompasses a total preoccupation with being here now, and not in the past or future, which is where many of our crippling and sleep-sucking thoughts lie.

In order to turn a chore like dishwashing into a mindfulness exercise, slow everything down; be mindful of your own breath and the sensations surrounding the dishwashing: the look and feel of the suds, the warmth of the water, the scent of your dishwashing soap. Focus exclusively on the task at hand and you will find that your anxious thoughts and worrying disappear. Essentially, you are crowding out competing thoughts and worries by over concentrating on the current activity.

In addition, try some moving meditation like tai chi or yoga, or even some simple stretching. A walk is also nice to do at night. Talk to your partner about how their day went, trade massages, read, listen to relaxing music, take a warm bath with Epsom salts for muscle relaxation—all of these can bridge the gap between the business of the day and the quiet rejuvenation of the night.

Try a nightly ritual of bathing to see what effect that has on your sleep. When I was younger I couldn't stand baths. I went decades without taking a single bath, preferring the quickness of a shower. I reasoned, *who has time to sit around and wait for a bathtub to fill with water, and what do you do in there anyway? Sitting in a bathtub has to be the ultimate in boring*, were my thoughts. Furthermore, why was it taking up so much valuable real estate in my bathroom?

And then I went through a period of amplified stress where I was searching for ways to decrease stress and improve my sleep. This is how I discovered the bathtub. The bathtub became my sanctuary, with bathtub accoutrements like candles, bath salts, essential oils, uplifting books, soothing music, and various decorations. I experimented with different bath salts and essential oils. Over time I developed the perfect nighttime ritual to calm me down and gently relax my body.

What I discovered was that plain old Epsom salts were the best bath salts to use for the bath. Epsom salts, otherwise known as magnesium sulfate, have a long reputation as being useful for sore muscles; but did you know it makes for a relaxing soak extraordinaire due to the same magnesium uptake of your body? Magnesium deficiency is very common in Americans and can contribute to many health issues as it is necessary for over 300 different reactions in your body. By soaking in magnesium sulfate, your body absorbs the minerals and raises your internal levels. During times of stress, magnesium is depleted, making an Epsom-salt bath a therapeutic strategy on multiple levels. Magnesium sulfate gently exfoliates your skin, leaving it soft, and relaxes your muscles, making it easier to go to sleep. As a bonus, Epsom salts are cheap and easily obtainable in any drug store or grocery store.

I like to add a few drops of essential oil to my bath. Lavender is a top favorite for its ability to soothe. One randomized, controlled study of patients in the intensive care unit (ICU) found that the inhalation of lavender essential oil reduced anxiety and increased sleep, as compared to the control group who had no intervention. People in the ICU typically do not sleep well for a variety of reasons and this simple, cheap, and effective sleep aid was shown to help. Another meta-analysis of inhaled lavender for the purposes of reducing anxiety and improving sleep looked at 15 different studies and concluded that lavender was a safe option for improving sleep. However, there are many other single and blended essential oils that can be tried for relaxation and sleep. Lavender is not the only one out there. The science of using essential oils for therapeutic benefits is called aromatherapy, and this area has exploded in popularity in the last few years.

As you get closer to getting into bed, or are in bed, a guided meditation, deep breathing exercises, hypnosis, or progressive-relaxation practices can help in the final nudge towards sleep.

Guided Meditations

I like guided meditations because, if you have trouble quieting your mind to meditate, having a soundtrack to guide you bypasses all of the angst you might have about not being able to even get started with a meditation. In a guided meditation, you will hear a voice, often accompanied by soothing music or nature sounds, lead you calmly into a meditative state. In terms of resources for guided meditations, there are many available on the internet, and some of them are free. In our technology-driven world today, you can easily download one onto your smartphone and listen to it tonight. You may need to listen to several before you narrow your choices down to one, as a particular voice or tone might be too annoying to you. Find one that works for you.

In terms of an upgraded, high-tech, guided meditation, there is a new device that joins soothing guided meditation, special lights, and sound, and can get you into the theta brain wave state within minutes. When I mentioned it in the previous chapter, I extolled its virtues for stress reduction, but it can also be used to help you fall asleep. The theta brain state is the meditative state, relaxed but not asleep, that normally takes a very experienced meditator to get into.

Theta states lead to higher levels of creativity, learning, and inspiration, and also can act as a prelude to actual sleep. You are already familiar with this state, as it is the dreamy, surreal feeling you get right before you fall asleep and after you open your eyes in the morning but are not yet awake.

When I discovered this technology, I knew I had to have it for myself. I tried it and discovered that it was the antidote to the two invisible enemies to beauty: stress and lack of sleep. Stress and lack of sleep are visible on your face and make you look older.

I now use this device daily, once in the afternoon for general stress reduction and creativity boost, and then before bed to make sure I can get my beauty sleep. I am so impressed with its results in me and in my patients that I also added it to my products available for sale on my website: it is called IAMFINE® Beauty Sleep System. However, if you are able to meditate effectively on your own, you don't need any device. Just meditate for the same results.

Progressive relaxation is also a great way to fall asleep. A guided, progressive relaxation will start at one end of your body and talk you through the melting, or relaxation, of each muscle group one by one. As muscle tension is often a sleep stealer, methodically relaxing each muscle group can help achieve total-body relaxation. When I was in medical school, I had a CD for progressive relaxation that I would actually listen to anytime in the day I had a break, not for going to sleep, but for reducing tension and anxiety. I found it quite helpful. Initially, however, it was shocking to discover that my muscles were so tight. Sometimes we are so stressed, we don't even realize how tight our muscles are; we can't even feel it.

Hypnotherapy can be an effective technique to utilize for better sleep. The best sleep aid I have ever used was an old-fashioned hypnotherapy audiotape from over 20 years ago titled "Sleep Like a Baby". Hypnotherapy uses the mind-body connection to enter an altered state of consciousness, or trance, where suggestions can be acted upon to improve health and instigate behavioral changes. There are many self-hypnosis CDs available today that are aimed at improving sleep, or you can make an appointment with a certified hypnotherapist who belongs to a national organization called the American Society of Clinical Hypnosis to have an in-person hypnotherapy session.

Deep breathing works very quickly for anxiety and is something that you can do right as you get into bed, or anytime during the day when you find yourself in a stressful situation. There are two important aspects to deep breathing, one of which is to breathe into your abdomen. Put your hands on your abdomen when you take a deep breath in and feel your abdomen rise. If you don't feel it rise, you are not breathing into your abdomen. Sometimes, this can take some time to learn. True story: when I first learned this I didn't even know your breath was *supposed* to go into your abdomen. I argued with the person who was trying to teach me how to breathe properly. Of course, as someone with lifelong asthma, I thought I knew all the tricks to breathing, including using my accessory muscles of respiration, when necessary, which are *not* located in the abdomen. People with asthma are pros at shallow chest breathing and may find deep, abdominal breathing difficult to get used to; but it is worth the effort.

Deep breathing also gets more oxygen into your cells. Cells use oxygen to make energy, repair DNA and other damaged structures in the cell. Increased oxygen also leads to more beautiful, healthy, rosy, and refreshed-looking skin. More oxygen translates into better skin and a healthier "color." Have you ever noticed how people who aren't feeling well have ashy or gray tones to their skin? Rosiness, or a red tint to the skin, is caused by increased oxygenation and is perceived as attractive and healthy.

Secondly, slow down your breathing and control it. One easy method is to inhale through your nose for a count of 5, hold for a count of 5, and exhale through your mouth for a count of 5. Alternatively, don't count at all and, in your mind, say on the breath in "sleep" or "peace" and literally breathe out the word "stress." It only takes 5-10 minutes of deep breathing to start feeling the results. Sometimes this is all someone needs to drift off into sleep.

Beauty Boost

- Power down one hour before bed
- Warm bath with Epsom salts
- Massage
- Yoga, Tai chi
- Guided meditation
- Hypnotherapy
- Progressive relaxation
- Deep breathing

Light Interference

Before the advent of electric light, people had a tendency to rise with the sun and go to sleep soon after sunset. This was a circadian biorhythm that worked with nature, as light, and its fading, acts on the pineal gland deep within the brain to control secretion of melatonin, a sleep-inducing neurotransmitter. By spending our days in artificial light, and the light from our computers, smartphones, iPads, and TVs, we have obliterated this natural pathway to falling asleep at night.

Light is turning out to be the most potent environmental signal that impacts the human circadian clock and may, therefore, play a role in perpetuating sleep deficiency. Accordingly, it has been the subject of much study globally as countries continue to mount evidence that artificial light and light-emitting technologies are wreaking havoc with sleep and subsequent alertness, health, safety, and performance in the daytime.

Studies have shown the effects of electrical light on secretion of melatonin at night, with effects being seen as longer times to fall asleep and lower levels of next-morning alertness. Surprisingly, this light-suppression effect on melatonin secretion in humans was more robust when the light is blue light, or the kind of light emitted from iPads, computers, and e-readers. A recent survey showed that 90% of Americans use an electronic device several nights a week within an hour of going to bed. No wonder we are a sleepless society!

In one study that evaluated people reading books the old-school way versus those reading books on an e-reader like an iPad before bed, some startling results were obtained. Now mind you, both the readers of printed books and the e-readers were being subjected to some form of artificial light in the time right before bed. Any light before bed, we have already been shown, has a negative impact on the secretion of melatonin at night.

What was found was that the e-readers had decreased sleepiness leading to taking a longer time to fall asleep, suppressed melatonin secretion, and less REM sleep, which is the deeply restorative part of the sleep cycle. They were also less alert than the printed-book readers the next morning. Specifically, the e-readers' circadian melatonin phase was one-and-a-half hours later than the print-book readers. There are clear biological ramifications to being exposed to this kind of light that is emitted from our electronic devices.

Is your iPad keeping you up at night too? The strong light-suppressing effects on melatonin are even more robust when the light emitted by iPads, computers, and smartphones (blue light) is considered. The research in humans has shown that light controls many physiological activities such as hormone secretion, heart rate, body temperature, alertness, and gene expression, making light an epigenetic modifier. Even more interesting, blue light, in particular, has the strongest effect on alertness, raising body temperature, suppressing melatonin, all physiological attributes that support NOT sleeping. In fact, blue light was found to suppress melatonin twice as long as green light. What this means is that your electronic device usage at night may be contributing to your sleep problems.

One way to decrease the light stimulation from your electronic devices at night is to download the free program from www.justgetflux.com . The F.lux program synchronizes your computer or other electronic device's screen with the sun so that as the sun goes down, your screen light "warms up," which means the blue light is cut and you can fall asleep more easily. I have this installed on my computer and it does make a difference. While this program adjusts to the sunset automatically, it also has a feature where you can turn it off if you have a project that needs to be worked on with full bright light.

Melatonin is a hormone secreted by the pineal gland, a pea-sized gland in the base of the brain. The ancient Greeks considered this gland to be the "seat of the Soul." Melatonin is secreted in response to the circadian rhythm and is the number one substance that puts you to sleep at night. When light fades, it is secreted and makes you long for your bed; when light creeps in your window in the morning, it shuts off its secretion and you wake up. Unfortunately, if you wake up in the middle of the night to visit the bathroom and turn on a light, your melatonin production is abruptly halted, making it that much harder to get back to sleep. All the blue light emitted from your many electrical devices like your computer also blocks melatonin production.

Melatonin has been shown to modulate immune defenses, body weight, and reproduction, and to have anticancer and anti-jet lag effects. In addition, it turns out that it is a super potent antioxidant and general anti-aging agent. Surprisingly, melatonin is found in high amounts in the skin and is felt to be biologically important to prevent the negative consequences of UV solar skin damage (skin aging and skin cancer). Well that's perfect for our discussion of beauty sleep! Is it the sleep, or is it the melatonin providing the beauty boost, or both?

Recent studies of melatonin expand on its therapeutic abilities in the skin. As it turns out, not only does the skin have receptors for melatonin made in the brain, it also manufactures its own melatonin. Not only does it act like a strong antioxidant, able to counteract the near constant barrage of free radicals formed from intrinsic and extrinsic aging, but it protects the DNA from genomic damage, acts like a cellular protectant, and reduces the MMP enzymes that destroy our collagen. The net result is that melatonin is a superb, skin-regenerative, beauty agent.

While you could take melatonin in supplement form, and I do recommend it when needed, there are ways to boost your body's own production:

- Avoid watching TV or using your computer or iPad in the hour or more before you go to bed.
- Make sure you expose your eyes to bright sun daily.
- Sleep in complete darkness; get rid of your nightlights and light-emitting clocks/alarm clocks in your room. Put blackout shades on your windows if they let in too much light at night. Or wear an eye mask when you sleep. Do NOT turn on a light to go to the bathroom at night. This will shut down your production of melatonin immediately. If it is unsafe to traverse your room to reach the bathroom, use a small nightlight that emits an orange, yellow, or red light.
- Get some sun in the morning. Only 10-15 minutes is necessary to instruct your body that day has arrived.
- Remove your clock from the bedroom. Not only does it emit light, but staring at the clock at 3:00 am and watching the minutes tick by with excruciating slowness, will not get you back to sleep.

Stimulation

Too much stimulation will keep you up at night. Caffeine from coffee, tea, or chocolate is an immediate culprit that comes to mind. Keep in mind that the half-life of caffeine is about 6 hours. That means, if you have 200 mg of caffeine in the morning, say at 9:00 am, 100 mg of caffeine is still in your system at 3:00 pm. And half of that, 50 mg of caffeine, is still percolating along in your bloodstream at 9:00 pm when it is time to start winding down for bed.

According to Starbuck's website, a 16-ounce cup of plain, Pike Place® Roast coffee contains 330 mg of caffeine. So, if you drank that at say, 3:00 pm, for a pick-me-up or to complete a fast approaching deadline, 165 mg of caffeine would still be around at 9:00 pm, which can be good or bad; good if you are still working, but it could possibly prevent you from sleeping, if you are ready to go to bed.

People have different abilities to metabolize caffeine. Some individuals are so sensitive to caffeine that one cup of coffee in the morning will keep them up all night. For sensitive people, it makes sense to avoid caffeine in order to get a good night's rest. Also watch the dark chocolate—it is surprisingly full of caffeine. In general, as the percentage of cacao increases, so does the caffeine content. On the other end of the spectrum is the group who can drink a cup of coffee right before bed and fall directly into a deep, restorative sleep.

Electromagnetic frequencies (EMFs) surround us day and night. Could they in any way be responsible for our current sleep crisis? EMFs are produced from wireless devices, smart meters, WiFi, Bluetooth, computers, and cell phones.

Some studies are showing a relationship between wireless devices and their emitted EMF and sleep. Citing longer times to get to sleep, less time in REM sleep, and more headaches, these studies suggest that we may not be getting the solid sleep that we need every night due to EMF fields.

Avoid sleeping with your cell phone next to your head or on your bedside table. Charge it in another room, if you are not using the alarm to wake up. If you are using your cell phone alarm to wake up, place the phone as far away from your head as possible. The same goes for your laptop and other electronic devices. Keep them all away from your head.

You can try an easy experiment in your home to see if Wi-Fi is contributing to your sleep problem. Simply switch off your Wi-Fi at night before you go to bed. This has been effective for many people. If you discover that you sleep better, then turning off the Wi-Fi before you go to bed just becomes another "light switch" to turn off.

You can also switch your house to Ethernet and get rid of the Wi-Fi altogether. This is what I have done and I can tell you, it has not only improved my sleep, but improved how I feel.

Watching a news channel before bed can also be entirely too stimulating. The human brain does not know the difference between something happening for real and something happening on TV or in a movie. Your body may still secrete adrenalin even if you are simply *watching* bad news on the TV or computer screen. The same goes for an action, horror, or violent movie that you watch before bed. Yet, many people watch the news in bed before they go to sleep and wonder why they are having a hard time falling asleep or staying asleep.

Noise at night, whether from the TV or outside traffic noise, can also affect sleep. This has been shown to be more highly associated with insomnia or sleep disturbances with anxious people. Ear plugs can be worn at night to shut out outside noises. On the other hand, some people find that white noise at night seems to help them sleep better. Experiment a little to see what works best for you.

Journaling or Expressive Writing

Sometimes we all have something we need to get off our chests at night. If we don't, we risk the chance of obsessing over it all night long. Journaling is a time-honored way to write down our thoughts so that we don't have to think about them all night long. Expressive writing, or writing a letter to a person who has wronged you or with whom you are having some kind of issue, is an exercise in which you write down your feelings and what you really want to tell that person, and really lay it all out there, and then burn or throw away the writing. It is not necessary to have the intended recipient read the letter. This exercise is for you; it has nothing to do with that person, and can be very cathartic.

Beauty Boost

- Cut down on caffeine
- Put the smart phone away from your head
- Turn off the Wi-Fi
- Don't watch the news before bed

Here are some sleep-specific tips:

- Start winding down an hour before you intend to go to bed. Do activities that support this such as yoga, meditation, tai chi, a walk, some mindless work around the house.

- Turn off the TV and computer.
- Start dimming lights at this time.
- Chamomile tea is a time-honored way to relax before bedtime.
- Certain relaxing and sedative herbs, such as hops, valerian, passionflower, and kava, can be taken before bed as a tea or in tincture form.
- Epsom-salt baths about an hour or two before bed is helpful to relax the muscles.
- Add some lavender essential oil drops to the bath for additional sleepy-time benefits.
- Listen to a relaxing CD of tranquil music, guided meditation, or some form of progressive relaxation.

Meditate, pray, journal. Find a way to release your worries to a higher power and listen for that still whisper that guides you along your path through life.

The Top Five Supplements for Sleep

- Melatonin: Melatonin is the sleep hormone released by your pineal gland when the lights go out. Melatonin is very helpful for sleep. Melatonin can induce more vivid dreaming and, in some people, nightmares and morning grogginess. If it has these effects for you, I would not recommend taking it.
- Hops (*Humulus lupulus*): Hops are a sedative herb and the bittering agent added to beer.
- Passionflower (*Passiflora incarnata*): Passionflower is an herb noted for its anxiolytic (anxiety busting) effects. It is also helpful for sleep.

- L-tryptophan: This amino acid is a precursor to serotonin (a neurotransmitter) and melatonin. Low levels of serotonin have been linked to insomnia, anxiety, and depression. It is best taken with pyridoxal 5 phosphate, the active form of B6, which is a necessary cofactor for the conversion of L-tryptophan.

- Valerian root (*valeriana officinalis*): This herb is the number-one herb used in the United States and Europe for inducing sleep. Notably, valerian root reduces the amount of time it takes to fall asleep and lacks a "hangover" effect the next morning. In a minority of people, it will induce the opposite effect: stimulation.

Due to the skin repair, collagen building, skin moisture retention, and beneficial effects on brain neurotransmitters and stress hormones, getting adequate sleep is the best and cheapest cosmetic out there! By utilizing some of the techniques in this chapter, you may be better able to get your beauty rest and see the increase in skin health in your mirror in the morning. Turn out the lights and get to bed already!

Applying the information

The Minimalist

- **Sleep more.** If you don't have trouble sleeping, but fall short of the recommended 8 hours per night, add 30 minutes more sleep per night until you reach that goal.

The Middle Way: Accompanying the above,

- Power down one hour before bed.
- Add F.lux to your devices to get rid of blue light.

The Beauty Buff: In Addition to All of the above,

- Turn off Wi-Fi or get Ethernet for your computers.
- Take sleep supplements if you have trouble sleeping.

CHAPTER NINE

Pure Products for Beauty

*"It's no longer enough to 'save the earth' because the earth is inside of us. We need to save ourselves."—**Dr. Fine***

AS A DOCTOR FOCUSED on environmental medicine, it struck me years ago that most of my patients with autoimmune disease, chronic fatigue, fibromyalgia, thyroid disease, hormonal imbalances, reproductive difficulties, and other chronic diseases were women. I pondered why that might be from an environmental-exposure perspective and wondered if it had to do with the sheer volume of chemicals women apply all over their bodies daily, sometimes multiple times per day.

This led me on a journey to investigate the very products women and their families use every single day and, much to my shock and dismay, I discovered that many of the ingredients in question were known or suspected to cause human health harm. This was my "aha" moment and what fuels my mission to educate physicians, consumers, and industry about toxic ingredients and their health consequences, as well as to provide guidance for companies intending to formulate safe products. To this end I am a frequent lecturer on the topic of toxicants in personal-care products and endocrine disruptors in everyday items at medical conferences around the U.S. and Europe.

I have also developed a four-module, online course aimed at consumers called "The Beauty Bluff" that explains exactly which ingredients you want to avoid in your personal-care products and why. The digital class can be found here: https://dr-anne-marie-fine.mykajabi.com/p/the-beauty-bluff .

Heavy metals, endocrine disruptors, carcinogens, allergens, and skin irritants are all present in our makeup and skin-care products and consumers have no way of knowing it. Since we are able to absorb certain compounds through our skin, it behooves us to take a look at the products we apply to our skin every day.

The skin's ability to absorb some of what we put on it should not come as a complete surprise to anybody. After all, we have transdermal patches for nicotine, hormones, pain medications, and more. Our skin turns out to be selectively permeable to what we put on it in terms of personal-care products. This has been established through many studies.

Compounds that penetrate the skin need to have a low molecular weight, an affinity for fat and, if it has skin-barrier impairment properties, so much the better for breaching the skin barrier. If certain substances are able to breach the skin, then they are carried by the blood throughout the body and can impart biological activity within the body. As personal care products are used for periods of months and years on a daily basis, and this effect is most likely not going to be acute and dramatic (i.e., no one is going to fall over dead after putting on a body product with questionable ingredients), we need to have better safety data for the ingredients that are being used.

Risk and safety assessment come into play here with most scientists stating that the "dose makes the poison," which comes from Paracelsus, a sixteenth-century physician, philosopher, botanist, and astrologer, and considered to be the father of toxicology. His statement refers to the fact that even a benign or "natural" substance such as water, when consumed in excess, can kill you. And that a very small amount of a substance considered a poison might not harm due to the tiny amount of the dose. This is the current state of toxicology today and the basis for which risk assessment is performed. In Paracelsus's time, there were relatively few "poisons" in the environment; certainly the 80,000 plus current chemicals being used in our world today did not exist back then.

Risk assessment usually looks for adverse effects of a certain compound over a range of high doses and, from there, extrapolates down to lower doses to establish health safety standards. The underlying assumption is that, as in Paracelsus's time, chemicals that are toxic at higher doses are much less risky at lower, real-world levels.

I think it is time to bring toxicology into the twenty-first century.

There is more to toxicity of materials than just the consideration of acute toxicity. In recent years, more attention has been focused on the cumulative effects of relatively small amounts of potentially harmful substances over a long time horizon of exposure. In addition, testing chemical mixtures, not just one at a time, which is the current standard of testing, would yield more real-world information about the ingredients. Are the effects additive, synergistic?

If there is only a little bit of lead in your home garden soil and "safe" amounts of arsenic in your water, it might not pose a very big risk to you in terms of cancer or other health effects. But say you are also being exposed to air pollution (as we all are) and live near industrial plants which have emissions (also within "safe" levels), use personal care products containing endocrine disruptors, eat food sprayed with pesticides, herbicides, and fungicides, have dental amalgams containing mercury and exposed to mercury from myriad other sources, and live across the street from a cell phone tower? Adding all of your exposures together, called the exposome, increases your risk for health harm, as these chemicals may act in concert on organs and tissues. Cumulative exposures to the many chemicals we are exposed to every day through ordinary items are what we should be studying for their health effects.

Furthermore, many of the endocrine disruptors have non-monotonic dose-response curves. That means a greater response is achieved at the lower doses and, when the amount goes up, the "toxicity" goes down. In other words, the dose does **not** make the poison.

Added to that is the fact that we are biochemically unique in our ability to metabolize or detoxify substances to which we are exposed. Certain variations in our liver-detoxification enzymes (single nucleotide polymorphisms, or SNPs) found in Phase I and Phase II Cytochrome P450 systems influence our ability to metabolize and excrete toxins. What that means is that certain people will detoxify certain substances better or worse than others, and that it is not possible to put everyone in the same category and assign the same risk assessments to them. I, for one, would like to see more environmental health studies stratify the participants on the basis of their detoxification SNPs and see what kind of results are obtained.

The skin also contains metabolizing enzymes and, likely, there is individual variation in this area as well. Furthermore, individuals may have epidermal-barrier dysfunction that permits more ingredients to penetrate the skin. Certainly, there are ingredients used in personal care products that are designed to be "penetration enhancers" which will drive other ingredients into the skin.

Personal care products represent the largest class of avoidable exposures to toxic ingredients, yet have not received the attention and awareness accorded to carcinogenic and toxic pollutants in air, water, and the home and workplace. Unlike those toxins, however, we can exercise control over what we put on our skin. Cosmetics and personal-care products are a modifiable threat to our health and a category with the widest range of emerging, alternative, safe products.

The FDA has no requirement for testing or approval before these products are marketed. There are also no mandates for label warnings identifying known allergens, carcinogens, or endocrine disruptors. This industry is self-regulated. While the European Union (EU) has adopted the Precautionary Principle in addressing potentially toxic chemicals in personal-care products before release, the United States looks for irrefutable proof of harm before recalling toxic ingredients.

Every day, at least 3 personal-care products are applied to the skin of infants and children. Women use 6 or more cosmetics and an average of 13 personal-care products daily containing over 100 different ingredients in total. Many women have applied over 100 different chemicals to their bodies before they even leave the house in the morning! Men use an average of 10 personal-care products per day. We are all exposed constantly and consistently to a sea of potentially problematic chemicals in the very products that we use to maintain our current standards of hygiene, cleanliness, and beauty.

This chapter will provide an overview of heavy metals, endocrine disruptors, overt and hidden problem ingredients, and skin allergens commonly found in personal-care products. Once armed with this eye-opening array of information, you can then check your own personal-care product labels and make a more informed decision on whether to keep it or choose another product for your personal use. Knowledge is definitely power here!

One caveat is that personal care products are only one source of toxicants going into your body. We take in many questionable ingredients and potentially harmful chemicals in our food supply, the air we breathe, the water we drink, and our home environment. For example, I will talk about phthalates in this chapter, a component of synthetic fragrances, but phthalates are also found in vinyl shower curtains, plug-in home air fresheners, laundry detergents, food wrappers, plastic toys, and your new car smell is partly the smell of phthalates off-gassing from your interior plastic parts. Please be aware that, while I recommend reducing phthalates, you must look at all sources of them, not just personal-care products.

Dr. Fine's Toxic Ten

1) Heavy metals (lead, mercury, cadmium)
2) Bisphenol A
3) Phthalates

4) Parabens

5) Triclosan, triclocarban

6) TEA, DEA, MEA

7) Formaldehyde releasers

8) Ethoxylated ingredients (1-4 dioxane and ethylene oxide as contaminants)

9) Fragrance and parfum

10) Petrolatum

Heavy Metals

Did you know lead is commonly found in lipsticks? The problem with this is that lipsticks can be ingested. While I believe it is nothing more than an urban myth that the average woman ingests seven pounds of lipstick over her lifetime, lipstick is one item of makeup that can and does wind up being eaten, merely by the lips' proximity to the mouth. I mean, there is a reason why lipstick and lip glosses need to be reapplied throughout the day.

What?!

The United States' own Food and Drug Administration (FDA) found lead in 100% of all lipsticks tested. Don't believe me? In an expanded study from 2010, they tested 400 lipsticks, the first ten results of which are listed below.

FDA Analyses of Lead in Lipsticks – Expanded Survey:

http://www.fda.gov/cosmetics/productsingredients/products/u cm137224.htm#expanded_survey

The results below for lead content in 400 lipsticks were obtained by Frontier Global Sciences, Inc., under a contract with the U.S.

Food and Drug Administration (FDA). The lipsticks were purchased from retail stores between February and July 2010.

Sample #	Brand	Parent company	Lipstick line Shade # Shade	Lot #a	Lead (Pb)b (ppm)
1	Maybelline	L'Oréal USA	Color Sensational 125 Pink Petal	FF205	7.19
2	L'Oréal	L'Oréal USA	Colour Riche 410 Volcanic	FE259	7.00
3	NARS	Shiseido	Semi-Matte 1005 Red Lizard	0KAW	4.93
4	Cover Girl Queen Collection	Procter & Gamble	Vibrant Hues Color Q580 Ruby Remix	9139	4.92
5	NARS	Shiseido	Semi-Matte 1009 Funny Face	9DLW	4.89
6	L'Oréal	L'Oréal USA	Colour Riche 165 Tickled Pink	FF224	4.45
7	L'Oréal	L'Oréal USA	Intensely Moisturizing Lipcolor 748 Heroic	FD306	4.41
8	Cover Girl	Procter & Gamble	Continuous Color 025 Warm Brick	9098	4.28
9	Maybelline	L'Oréal USA	Color Sensational 475 Mauve Me	FF201	4.23
10	Stargazer	Stargazer	Lipstick 103 c	180808	4.12

Lead levels are cumulative, and applying lead-containing cosmetics several times a day or every day can potentially add up to significant exposure levels, especially with lip products that can and do wind up being ingested due to sheer proximity to the mouth and the unavoidability of having your lips touch the food you bite into. Some surveys say women apply lipstick up to 2-14 times a day. Pregnant and nursing mothers are a vulnerable population because lead passes through placenta and human milk and can affect the fetus's or infant's developments. Of particular note, lead is an environmental neurotoxicant known to interfere with brain development, and the association between even **low levels of lead in the blood of children and reduced IQ scores is robust.**

From the Centers for Disease Control's website:

> "Protecting children from exposure to lead is important to lifelong good health. No safe blood lead level in children has been identified. Even low levels of lead in blood have been shown to affect IQ, ability to pay attention, and academic achievement. And effects of lead exposure cannot be corrected. The most important step parents, doctors, and others can take is to **prevent lead exposure before it occurs.**" https://www.cdc.gov/nceh/lead/acclpp/blood_lead_levels.htm

According to a University of California study, women apply lipstick from to 2-10 times a day. While a single application of lipstick will not make you ill, the fact that women apply it several times a day, and that they do this over a lifespan, results in an accumulation of lead. This same study, published in *Environmental Health Perspectives*, found, in addition to lead, **chromium, cadmium, aluminum, and manganese,** and other heavy metals of concern, in the same lip products (8 lipsticks and 24 lip glosses).

These heavy metals are not added intentionally to lip products through the manufacturing process, but instead are impurities or contaminants in the pigments used to add color. This means you will not find them listed anywhere on the label, making it impossible to know if your lipstick is safe. When you ask the sales person of a lipstick or color makeup company, they are in no way trained to be able to answer the question thoughtfully or truthfully as they are so far removed from the mining/sourcing of the pigments that their raw material supplier used. They will truthfully (and perhaps indignantly) say, "Of course we don't add lead to our products." Lead is not added to products.

Because cosmetics are not the only way lead might accumulate in the body, women who are planning to conceive, pregnant, or nursing might be very motivated to seek out personal-care products with low or no lead levels detected. This will help to minimize the amount of lead they are passing on to their children, thereby protecting intelligence levels and behavior.

Numerous other studies have raised the same kind of concern with heavy metal contamination of makeup. In the peer-reviewed journal *Contact Dermatitis*, it was found that 75% of the eyeshadow colors contained more than five parts per million of at least one of the heavy metals lead, cobalt, nickel, chromium and arsenic. This particular study was concerned with the sensitizing aspects of metals found in the products, not the potentially toxic effects. Personal-product ingredients may be allergenic in an individual, completely aside from any toxicity issues, which we will discuss later in this chapter.

The presence of heavy metals in makeup is mainly due to the contamination of the pigments used in the products; they are product impurities. They are not added intentionally, nor are they listed on the label, making it difficult to know if the products you are using are contaminated or not. The problem with heavy metals is that they can accumulate in the body over time and cause health issues. While toxins are tested one at a time to determine whether or not there are safety concerns at a particular level, we are exposed to multiple toxins at a time from numerous sources over a lifespan, making it nearly impossible to point the finger at any one product or source. This is why it makes sense to limit your exposure. In the case of personal-care products, if we know which products are less contaminated with heavy metals or other undesirable ingredients, we can make better choices for us and our families.

Endocrine-Disrupting Chemicals (EDCs)

Before we begin, let's start with a definition of "endocrine disruptor." Your endocrine system refers to your total hormone system consisting of thyroid, adrenals, pancreas, reproductive organs, hypothalamus, and pineal gland. An endocrine disruptor is a substance which interferes with the normal hormone activity of a certain gland in the body. Often, this happens at very low doses, which is why the existence of endocrine-disrupting chemicals (EDCs) in our environment pose such a threat to our health. It turns the old "dose makes the poison" argument on its head, as hormone activity itself occurs at extremely low levels of hormones.

According to the Endocrine Society, the most active organization devoted to research on hormones and the clinical practice of endocrinology, "exposure to EDCs during fetal development and puberty plays a role in the increased incidences of reproductive disease, endocrine-related cancers, behavioral and learning problems including ADHD, infections, asthma, and perhaps obesity and diabetes in humans."

And speaking of reproductive diseases, these are some of the most common problems that are presented today. From a naturopathic, integrative, and holistic perspective, the reproductive system is one of the first to be comprised when the body is not at optimal performance because the reproductive system is not necessary for day-to-day function. This is why women who are starving or overtraining so often will lose their periods—their body knows it is not the best time to have a baby, so resources are conserved and not expended on that monthly process.

Thyroid disease is also rampant today. Much of thyroid disease is linked to chemicals and toxins in the environment, such as the endocrine disruptors, perchlorate, pesticides, mercury, phthalates, and bisphenol A.

Most thyroid problems are hypothyroidism, making it hard to lose weight and feel good. By learning which chemicals in our environment are contributing to poor thyroid function, we can avoid them and improve our thyroid function, which can lead to weight loss and energy gain.

Many of my patients have been able to improve their thyroid function through addressing environmental toxicants, which includes choosing to buy clean personal-care products. This has been a game changer for them and they get their zest for life back and start feeling good again!

A 2015 economic analysis of the European Union found that exposure to endocrine-disrupting chemicals likely costs €157 billion a year in actual healthcare costs and lost earning power. Included in this analysis are two of the EDCs that are associated with personal-care products: phthalates and bisphenol A (BPA).

Recently, a similar report came out for the United States that puts the annual costs of healthcare costs and lost wages at $340 billion per year, more than that of the European Union due to a less strict regulatory environment in the U.S. Of that, about $50 billion is due to BPA alone. It's clear that endocrine disruptors are harming our health and costing us dearly.

The expert panel in the EU study identified a 40-69% probability of phthalate exposure causing 53,900 cases of obesity in older women with a €15.6 billion price tag attached. Separately, in those women who further develop new-onset diabetes, €607 million of additional costs must be considered. Prenatal bisphenol A (BPA) exposure was identified to have a 20-69% probability of causing 42,400 cases of childhood obesity, with associated lifetime costs of €1.54 billion. That's an enormous impact!

In the U.S. version of the same cost analysis of endocrine disruptors, 2/3 of the health effects and costs were related to flame retardants, or polybrominated diphenyl ethers (PBDEs). Thankfully, this is not something we have to worry about in personal-care products and efforts are underway to revise regulations involving flame retardants in our home furnishings, although it will take years to get them out. In the meantime, mattresses, couches, seat cushions, electronics, cars, and airplanes all are treated with flame retardants.

Children's pajamas are also treated with flame retardants, which is not a great idea as toxicants can migrate out of the materials they are put into and move into us. Researchers found the chemicals used as flame retardants were to blame for:

- Thyroid disruption
- Early-onset puberty
- Cognitive problems
- Delayed mental and physical development

EDCs are commonly found in food and food packaging, plastics, and plastic bottles and containers, furniture, toys, carpeting, some building materials, cosmetics, and other personal care products. As virtually all chemical research focuses on one chemical substance at a time, it is hard to know what the exposure to complex mixtures of hundreds of EDCs might be doing to our bodies. In reality, no one is exposed to just one chemical at a time.

Currently, biomonitoring activities by scientists at the Centers for Disease Control measure pesticides and other chemicals in the bodies of Americans every few years. In the most recent study, CDC tested for 212 chemicals, including 44 pesticides, and found most of them in the bodies tested. One of them, a breakdown product of DDT, a pesticide banned over 40 years ago, was found in 99% of Americans tested, demonstrating that some of these chemicals are persistent in the environment and do not break down over time, eventually finding their ways into our bodies through our food supply. This should shock you because some chemicals which were finally found to be too toxic to use anymore and were subsequently banned in the 1970s are still found in people today. These are called "persistent organic pollutants" and are a special class of problematic substances that hang around in our environment for seemingly forever.

Studies have shown that newborns are being born with hundreds of chemicals already in their bodies, indicating that the potential for health risks starts *in utero*. These chemicals include pesticides, heavy metals, flame retardants, and various EDCs. The research of how these chemicals impact human growth and development is still in its infancy, but animal studies have already sounded an alarm on the unintended side effects of our modern environment on our health and the health of our unborn children.

While nearly all of the research involving chemicals and their effects in the body are done one chemical at a time, it is incumbent upon scientists to begin studying the mixtures of chemicals that we all have in our bodies starting in the womb. Are the effects additive or are the effects synergistic? Do they interact with each other?

For example, it is known that exposure to certain chemicals during fetal development can increase the risk of adverse health effects, but little is known about how many different chemicals are actually found in pregnant women, let alone their combined health effects.

One study tested pregnant women in the United States for 71 different chemicals and found a median of 50 in each pregnant woman. Certain chemicals, such as polychlorinated biphenyls or PCBs (banned since the 1970s but persistent in the environment), organochlorine pesticides, bisphenol A (BPA), flame retardants, car exhaust, phthalates, and perchlorate (an ingredient found in rocket fuel) were detected in 99-100% of the pregnant women tested.

So, what are some of these EDCs? Among chemicals known to be EDCs are PCBs, dioxins, solvents, phthalates, BPA, organophosphate and organochlorine pesticides, and polybrominated diphenyl ethers (PBDEs), otherwise known as flame retardants.

While these may sound like the answers to a chemistry quiz, these compounds are very present, even ubiquitous, in our environment. PCBs and dioxins are found in our diet (animal foods), solvents are found in dry cleaning solution and degreasers, phthalates and BPA are in personal-care products discussed separately below, pesticides are found in our diet, but also in public places that spray for pests, and PBDEs are flame retardants found in upholstered furniture, mattresses, baby seats, electronics, cars, and airplanes.

The four main EDCs that are found in personal-care products are bisphenol A, phthalates, parabens, and triclosan, and we will talk about them in the next section.

Bisphenol A

Bisphenol A (BPA) is a great example of the difficulty and controversy of assessing environmental health hazards. Edward Charles Dodds, a British medical researcher at the University of London, identified the estrogenic properties of BPA in the mid-1930s while researching synthetic estrogen. He found the estrogenic properties of BPA rather weak and continued his search until he found a more powerful estrogenic substance, diethylstilbestrol (DES), which he subsequently brought to market with disastrous consequences as it promoted cancer in daughters born to mothers who took it. Given its origins, it is not surprising that BPA has been found to be an endocrine disruptor and linked to cancer.

BPA was dropped as a drug, but enjoyed a brilliant career in plastics. It is considered a high throughput chemical, with commercial applications in epoxy resin and liners for metal equipment, piping, steel drums, and the interior of food cans, as well as adhesives to lay flooring and seal teeth. In the 1950s, it was made into polycarbonate material used in electronics, safety equipment, automobiles, and plastic food containers as well as the ubiquitous plastic water bottles. It is also found in children's toys, sippy cups, infant formula (leaching from the can lining), baby bottles, IV tubing, canned foods including sodas, that glossy coating on sales register receipts, and even in some prescription medications as a coating. Over six billion pounds of BPA are produced yearly.

BPA has also contaminated human tissue. The NHANES III study demonstrates widespread human exposure to BPA in 93% of urine samples from humans 6 years and older. The same study revealed that infants (0-6 months) fed formula from plastic bottles had up to ten times the BPA in their urine than breast-fed infants. This is significant because even the breast-fed infants had BPA in their urine, likely from mom's breast milk, meaning mom is already contaminated even before she breastfeeds.

BPA has been found in breast milk, amniotic fluid, cord blood, serum, and saliva. The Endocrine Society, a professional scientific organization devoted to hormone research, warns that bisphenol A and other endocrine-disrupting chemicals (EDC) "have effects on male and female reproduction, breast development and cancer, prostate cancer, neuroendocrinology, thyroid, metabolism and obesity, and cardiovascular endocrinology."

Over two hundred scientific studies have demonstrated that very low doses of BPA correlate to cancers, especially breast and prostate, impaired immune function, early onset of puberty, obesity, diabetes, and hyperactivity. The median level of BPA in humans exceeds the level proven to cause damage in animal studies. BPA is also associated with oxidative stress and inflammation in postmenopausal women.

A recent study examined BPA exposure to rats in utero and discovered that, at relevant human exposures, BPA altered mammary glands embryonically to result in cancer later in life. This could help explain how breast cancer rates have skyrocketed starting in the twentieth century.

How do we avoid BPA in our environment? The first rule of environmental medicine is avoidance. If you avoid the chemical in the first place, you won't have to detoxify it later. Does avoidance work?

According to a recent pilot study of female college students, it does work. At California Polytechnic State University in San Luis Obispo, CA, two groups of women participated in a BPA-avoidance study. One group received face-to-face counseling on how to avoid BPA exposure and was given BPA-free cosmetics and personal-care products, glass food-storage containers, and advised to eat only organic foods; the other group received only generalized information about BPA. After only three weeks, the women who had received the BPA-free items and face-to-face counseling had reduced levels of BPA in their bodies. As a bonus, they lost significant weight. Yep, plastic makes you fat because it is an endocrine disruptor and affects your pancreatic output of insulin as well as your thyroid gland, your master regulator of metabolism.

Choose glass whenever possible for eating, storing food, and drinking. We all have kitchens full of plastic containers with lids for food storage and leftovers. Some of us drink out of plastic glasses, even in the home, and nearly all of us drink water from plastic water bottles when we are out of the home. Plastic sports and hiking water bottles also abound in our personal environment.

Glass Tupperware-style containers have cropped up in the marketplace. Indeed, that is what I use exclusively in my kitchen for food storage. These are easily available at Costco, Amazon, and Target. Never microwave your food in plastic either, as the heat facilitates transfer of plastic into your foods.

While many "green" companies have jumped on the BPA-free bandwagon, brandishing their BPA-free labels on anything from baby sippy cups, to plastic water bottles, the new studies reveal that the BPA substitutes are many times just as bad, or even worse, in their estrogenic properties. So, don't be fooled by BPA-free marketing claims. Beware the Regrettable Substitutions! Regrettable Substitutions are the replacement chemicals used when a substance, like BPA, is found to be problematic. Unfortunately, the substitutions themselves are not properly vetted, and often wind up being from the same chemical family, and capable of the same health effects. For example, BPA substitutions BPS and BPF have the same problems as BPA.

Just use glass. Innovators are coming out with glass storage containers and water bottles, often cleverly supported by a netting of a soft plastic that does not come in contact with the contents, but prevents the glass from breaking in a fall. I have seen this on baby bottles as well.

Stainless steel water containers have also come out on the market, which can be used as an alternative to plastic. These containers don't have the breakage worries and may even be lighter than the glass options.

Canned foods also have BPA in their liners. While some manufacturers have changed to BPA-free liners, the same problems arise as in the BPA substitutes not being shown to be an improvement. Avoid canned food whenever possible.

In one eye-opening experiment done at the Harvard School of Public Health, two groups of people were asked to eat one serving of soup per day. In one group, the soup was canned, in the other group, the soup was homemade. After only 5 days, the canned soup eating group had more than 1,000% more BPA in their urine than the homemade soup eaters. And that was only one source of BPA over a short time frame!

Thermal cash register receipts are also tainted with BPA. One enlightening study demonstrated that the combination of French fries, hand sanitizer, and handling of thermal receipts resulted in an even higher amount of BPA in blood and urine, than handling of the receipt alone.

The use of hand-sanitizer and other skin-care products including hand lotion, cremes, and sunscreens contain ingredients that are penetration enhancers such as isopropyl myristate and propylene glycol can facilitate up to 100 times the absorption of other ingredients, such as BPA. In the study above, it was found that using a hand sanitizer before touching the thermal receipt, and then eating French fries in a fast food restaurant, resulted in a much higher concentration of BPA in the blood and urine than touching the thermal receipt with a dry hand (no hand-sanitizer being used).

This study illustrates two issues: the issue of penetration enhancers added to personal care products which greatly facilitate the admission of other dermal ingredients into the body, and the fact that thermal receipts contain BPA which transfers to our fingers in mere seconds.

Given the sheer number of receipts we might get in an average day from the coffee shop, grocery store, gas station, bank, etc., you might want to think about informing the cashier that you don't want your receipt. Obviously, for high-ticket items and things you may want to return, it is better to keep the receipt.

Phthalates

Phthalates, chemicals with potential estrogenic action, are mainly used as plasticizers (making plastics more flexible) and are present in a wide range of consumer products such as polyvinyl chloride flooring, shower curtains, detergents, plastic clothing, pharmaceuticals, IV bags and tubing, children's toys, and personal-care products. Phthalates also occur in our diet due to leaching into our food via plastic packaging including water bottles. In cosmetics, they are found in deodorants, nail polishes, perfumes, and other products that contain fragrances, which are most of them.

In humans, phthalates have been found in blood, urine, saliva, amniotic fluid, breast milk and cord (fetal) blood. Their adverse effects are due to their endocrine-disrupting ability and include effects on reproduction such as sperm damage, early-onset puberty in women, anatomical anomalies of the reproductive tract, infertility, and adverse outcomes of pregnancy.

The Environmental Working Group (EWG) found phthalates in 75% of 72 personal-care products tested. One hundred percent of fragrances tested positive for phthalates in the same study. None of the products containing phthalates included it on the label. Fragrance is protected as a trade secret and not required to be listed on the label. In the United States, "fragrance" is simply a trade name for between 100 and 300 different scent chemicals, but phthalates are used as scent carriers or fixatives and that explains their presence in fragrances.

The EU bans carcinogenic and mutagenic chemicals and reproductive toxins from cosmetic products. The phthalates benzyl butyl phthalate (BBP), dibutyl phthalate (DBP), and diethyhexyl phthalate (DEHP) were banned in 2003 due to their classification as toxic to reproduction. Despite this regulation, cosmetic companies often use these chemicals in markets that do not prohibit them, including that of the United States.

To avoid phthalates in your personal-care products, seek out the products that do not contain "fragrance" or "parfum." These terms on a product label will alert you to the high probability of phthalates being in your product. Phthalates will never be listed as "phthalates" on a product, since they are contained or subsumed under the category of fragrance, which usually means dozens of unidentified ingredients protected under trade-secret agreements.

use

High quality essential oils do not contain phthalates and their scent is from the actual botanical plant mass from which the oils are made.

Don't use

Home plug-in fragrances are also a huge source of phthalates in the home. I am always surprised to see these everywhere, in bathrooms, living rooms, dorm rooms, and apartments. Spray fragrances are also very popular to mask unpleasant smells in the home. The key here is that they can only "mask" the odor. It is far better to actually get rid of the odor. Opening the windows and airing out the house daily, taking out the garbage, and certain house plants are much safer ways to create fresh air in the home without having to resort to synthetic fragrances called "Spring Air" being constantly pumped into your living spaces. Who wants to breathe in additional chemicals, especially when those chemicals include benzene, a known carcinogen, styrene, and formaldehyde?

Nail polish notoriously contains the toxic trifecta of toluene, formaldehyde, and phthalates. In recent years, the manufacturers have been voluntarily removing one or more of these from their nail polishes. However, a disturbing study of 25 nail polishes labeled non-toxic recently found that many polishes that claimed to be toxin-free contained one, two, or all three of the toxins. So, what's a girl to do?

One solution is to use a water-based nail polish. Another solution is to search out clean-scoring nail polishes on the Skin Deep and Think Dirty databases described later in this chapter. Some large and well-known nail polish purveyors have also made significant progress in removing these carcinogens and reproductive toxins from their formulations. Unfortunately, the replacement chemical to give the polish flexibility, triphenyl phosphate or TPHP, is turning out to be another suspected endocrine disruptor. This nail polish chemical doubles as a furniture fire retardant! In animal studies it contributes to type-2 diabetes and fat accumulation—this is not something we women need.

My favorite solution of all is just not to wear nail polish. I can count on one hand the number of times I have had a mani or a pedi. Natural and healthy nails go with anything and require no upkeep or financial investment. You can maintain your nails, cuticles, and address your calluses at home. But if you do enjoy the creative expression of nail polish, look for safer options. There are also organic nail salons coming on the market.

Parabens

Parabens have been shown to be estrogenic in vivo and in vitro and have been detected in human breast-tumor tissue, cord blood, and breast milk. Studies have demonstrated the ability of parabens to penetrate human skin, and act as endocrine disrupters, changing our normal male and female hormones, as well as other hormones. They inhibit our ability to detoxify estrogen, which suggests that parabens may also indirectly enhance estrogen effects through elevation of free estradiol levels, and recent studies have reported that they may cause DNA damage.

Parabens are nearly ubiquitous in personal-care products such as deodorant, shampoo, conditioner, and moisturizers, although paraben-free alternatives do exist. In one study, 99% of cosmetics tested contained parabens. In addition, parabens can be found in foods.

Recently, their potential endocrine-disrupting effects have raised concerns about their safety and their potential effects as emerging pollutants leading to the regulation of the presence of parabens in commercial products by national and trans-national organizations.

Parabens have been at the center of a controversy about whether or not they cause breast cancer since 2004, when intact parabens were found in breast-cancer tumors, and the research continues to grow. A U.S. analysis found that 99% of people tested had methyparaben in their bodies. European studies show much the same, with one Spanish study showing 100% of pregnant women's and children's urine contained parabens.

In a study involving breasts removed during mastectomies for breast cancer, the breasts were sectioned in four parts, from the armpit to the breastbone, to investigate paraben content. Perhaps not surprisingly, 99% of the breast samples contained at least one paraben; 60% contained all 5 parabens. Paraben content was not correlated to tumor location as these samples were unaffected breast tissue from a breast-cancer-afflicted breast. However, paraben content in the lateral parts of the breast were higher in users of underarm deodorant and antiperspirants. This folds in with previous conclusions in studies aiming to link the use of underarm cosmetics with paraben accumulation in the outer parts of the breast that lie closest to the underarm.

What I found fascinating and a little disturbing is that, compared to the original study using actual **breast tumor samples** from the 1980s that were detailed in the 2004 study that found parabens in breast cancer, this study of **NON-cancerous breast tissues** showed quantities of parabens that were **400% higher** than the cancerous tumors of the 1980s. Although neither study ascertained where the parabens were coming from, it would seem that, a few decades later, the amounts have risen considerably.

Since there are some 160 xenoestrogens (substances that act like estrogen in the body) that may be involved in breast cancer development, looking at combinations of them may yield the most information about their health effects in the body, rather than just trying to blame one of them. This is where the research needs to go. We need to get out of the testing dogma that tests one chemical at a time—it's not a real-life situation.

In the meantime, more recent studies have concluded that parabens have the ability to *enable multiple hallmarks of cancer progression* and have multiple influences on molecular pathways that involve the hormone system. What this means is that the traditional test to determine if a substance is carcinogenic usually looks at the substance's ability to **initiate** cancer. But there are multiple steps along the way, which must be met, for that cancer to progress. And these recent studies demonstrate that parabens enable four of six of the basic hallmarks of cancer progression, one of two of the emerging hallmarks, and one of two of the enabling characteristics. This finding deserves more study as it can change the framework in which parabens are viewed from a toxicological perspective.

While parabens are classified as having very weak estrogenic activity, the newer research reveals that, with a high enough concentration of one or perhaps a combination of parabens, the estrogen-binding capability is the same as our body's own estrogen. Perhaps the question should not be how weak is the estrogen-binding capability, but what is the concentration of parabens found in the target tissue at which level the "weak" estrogen-binding characteristic can be overcome?

If we study parabens in combination with other estrogen-like chemicals in the breast tissue, would we get more clarity on the origins of breast cancer?

Triclosan

When I was growing up there was only "soap," as in bar soap; then came the advent of liquid soaps in all their colorful-plastic-bottle glory. Subsequently, beginning in the 1990s antibacterial soaps became all the rage. It is estimated that about 75% of liquid hand soap and 30% of bar soap now contain triclosan

Triclosan was first registered as a pesticide in 1969, but is now commonly known as an antimicrobial product found in soap, detergent, toothpaste, fabric, facial tissue, clothes, paper products, and toys. It is also used as a preservative in numerous products, such as building materials, polyethylene, polypropylene, polyurethane, and carpeting. Widespread in consumer products, it is now almost ubiquitous in human urine. The Centers for Disease Control (CDC) found triclosan in 75% of human beings tested. It has also been found in human breast milk and infant cord blood.

Studies on triclosan indicate that it is an endocrine disruptor, specifically targeting thyroid function. And, boy, is thyroid disease rampant in my patient population. There are also growing concerns related to microbial antibiotic resistance.

At this time, after looking at data from 30 different studies, the FDA has no evidence that triclosan is any more effective than soap and hot water to deter transference of disease.

Basic handwashing with hot water and soap is so central to maintenance of good health, that adding an antibacterial ingredient, such as triclosan, isn't even necessary or effective, especially given its potential for endocrine disruption.

Triclosan is already regulated in Europe, Canada, and Japan. Recently, in the U.S., the FDA banned the use of triclosan in antiseptic formulations, although it is still permitted in other products such as toothpaste. Read the label to see if is in your products.

I teach avoidance to my patients for the reason that it works. As a case in point, there was a study done with teen girls in California where the girls were given personal-care products and makeup free of phthalates, parabens, triclosan, and benzophenone-3. At the end of **only three days**, the urine samples showed that methyl-paraben decreased by 43.9%, propyl-paraben decreased by 45.4%, phthalates decreased by 27.4%, and triclosan decreased by 35.7%. That was a significant drop over just a three-day period.

Hidden Toxins and Allergens

The lack of total disclosure on product labels is an insidious component of the personal-care product issue. It is important to know which compounds are designed to release formaldehyde, are contaminated by carcinogens, or might be allergens.

TEA, MEA and DEA

The ethanolamine compounds: triethanolamine (TEA), monoethanolamine (MEA), and diethanolamine (DEA) and are used frequently in personal-care products as foaming agents and emulsifiers.

DEA is a possible human carcinogen and restricted in some countries from being used in personal-care products. It is also irritating to the skin. In laboratory studies, exposure to these substances has been shown to cause liver cancers and precancerous changes in the skin and thyroid gland.

The more worrisome aspect to these compounds is their potential reaction with other ingredients in a formulation to form probable human carcinogenic nitrosamines, which are never listed on a label since it would be a contaminant or unintended consequence. Since we use so many personal-care products daily, and for decades at a time, the potential for harmful effects persists. Look for labels that don't contain these ingredients

On the label look for:

- Cocamide DEA
- Cocamide MEA

- DEA-Cetyl Phosphate
- DEA Oleth-3 Phosphate
- TEA-Lauryl Sulfate
- Triethanolamine

Formaldehyde Releasers

Formaldehyde is actually a great preservative. After all, the human cadavers we used in anatomy lab in medical school were preserved with formaldehyde and it worked great. Of course, we all wore gas masks in order to avoid the respiratory problems that came along with breathing formaldehyde.

According to the Occupational Safety & Health Administration (OSHA) website:

"Formaldehyde is a known cancer-causing substance. Exposure to formaldehyde can also cause:

- Eye irritation and damage, including blindness
- Nose irritation, including bloody noses
- Skin sensitivity, rashes, and itching
- Breathing difficulties, such as coughing and wheezing"

In 2011, The National Toxicology Program also listed formaldehyde as a known human carcinogen in their *Twelfth Report on Carcinogens*. As a known carcinogen, it is not permitted to be used as an ingredient in personal-care products above the approved level of 0.2% according to the cosmetic industry's own regulatory group.

However, formaldehyde-releasing preservative systems that preserve products by slowly releasing formaldehyde into the product over time, *are* used in personal-care products. This is a very clever way to get around formaldehyde's bad reputation because the word formaldehyde need not appear on the label.

The health concerns with formaldehyde releasers include direct toxic effects and contact dermatitis (discussed farther along in this chapter) for many users. Twenty percent of all cosmetic products, including 17% of stay-on products and 27% of wash-off products, contain formaldehyde releasers. These ingredients include:

- quaternium-15
- dimethyl-dimethyl (DMDM)
- hydantoin
- imidazolidinyl urea
- diazolidinyl urea
- 2-bromo-2-nitropropane-1,3-diol (bronopol)
- sodium hydroxylmethylglycinate.

So, if these ingredients are present on the label, it is an indication that the product will have formaldehyde in it.

Interestingly enough, a well-known mass marketer of a popular baby shampoo that traded on their slogan "no more tears" very recently reformulated its iconic shampoo to take out the formaldehyde-releasing preservative system. Having personally witnessed plenty of tears when I tried that brand on my babies, I suspect the formaldehyde was the culprit.

Speaking of hair products containing formaldehyde, hair straightening (also called keratin treatment) and smoothing products such as the Brazilian Blowout have been called out due to their use of this substance, while brazenly labeling their product as formaldehyde-free. Due to the respiratory and other effects of being around the airborne formaldehyde, various regulatory agencies became involved to help sort it all out. To this day, the product remains available despite the warnings dispensed. Salon workers have complained about losing their hair, headaches, breathing difficulties, and fatigue with some workers unable to continue to work. Those who are sensitive to certain chemicals, pregnant or breastfeeding, or currently have cancer or wish to prevent any exposure to superfluous toxins, should avoid this kind of product.

I frequented a non-toxic salon that I thought would prevent me from ever having to experience the keratin treatment (hair straightening) toxic environment, but I was mistaken. One day I was having my hair done, and my eyes, throat, and lungs started burning. I couldn't think of what the problem might be, but I asked my stylist if keratin straightening products were used there. Much to my surprise, she said YES! Really? It's disheartening that even the non-toxic salons allow these products to be used. When I could no longer open my eyes, my stylist moved me as far away from the formaldehyde fumes as she could; but I no longer go to that salon.

In the same way formaldehyde straightens the hair, it also straightens fabrics. Those items of clothing that promise no ironing and look as if they could stand up and walk out of the store with you because they are so stiff and straight, also have formaldehyde embedded in the fabric.

I would much prefer to avoid them altogether in my personal care products. Why are carcinogens allowed in our personal care products at *any* level, anyway?

Ethoxylated Ingredients (1,4-dioxane and ethylene oxide contaminants)

1, 4-dioxane and ethylene oxide are carcinogenic contaminants found in many personal-care products, including organic ones. While you will never see it on a label because it is a by-product of a chemical reaction in a formulation, this compound easily penetrates the skin. Fortunately, it is easy to avoid if you look on the label and see ingredients with the following names:

- Sodium laureth sulfate
- Polyethylene
- Polyethylene glycol (PEG)
- Polyoxyethylene
- Polysorbate
- Or any ingredient with "xynol," "ceteareth," or "oleth."

These ingredients are ethoxylated, meaning they have been chemically reacted with ethylene oxide to form the new ingredients. This chemical process leaves the byproducts, 1,4-dioxane and ethylene oxide; both carcinogens.

Fragrance

Fragrance may epitomize the cosmetic industry's regulatory and labeling issues for the uninformed consumer. The term "fragrance" is designed to conjure romantic images, but what does anyone really know about any specific fragrance? Fragrance is considered a proprietary ingredient, is exempt from labeling requirements, and, although labeled as one item, usually contains numerous compounds.

Even the term "scent-free" may imply the use of fragrance to cover up an inherent odor.

In 2007, the American Contact Dermatitis Society named "fragrance" the Allergen of the Year. More recently, the Campaign for Safe Cosmetics and the Environmental Working Group examined 17 name-brand fragrances for semi-volatile organic compounds, VOCs, and synthetic musk. The study revealed a total of 38 undisclosed chemicals, including sensitizers, endocrine disruptors, carcinogens, and neurotoxins. Some ingredients were found to perpetuate skin damage. Numerous ingredients were found to lack rigorous toxicity data. The irony is that fragrance is marketed as "sexy" when, in fact, its toxicity may contribute to breast cancer, early puberty, poor genital development, skin disease, and allergy. All in all, not a very sexy picture.

Fragrance also contains phthalates, which were previously described.

Petrolatum

Petrolatum, or petroleum jelly, is a product derived from petroleum. It is a distinctive jelly-like substance used for soothing dry skin. Petrolatum, since it is derived from crude oil byproducts, may be contaminated with polyaromatic hydrocarbons, which are reasonably anticipated to be human carcinogens. It also prevents the skin from breathing due to its high skin-occlusive ability.

Allergens

Certain ingredients in personal-care products may cause allergic reactions, or allergic contact dermatitis, in susceptible individuals.

Allergic contact dermatitis results in a red, itchy rash or bumps in an area in direct contact with an offending substance. Unlike the toxins listed above whose insidious accumulation and contribution to total body burden may cause a health problem down the road, an allergic reaction is much more obvious and sudden, normally leading to a swift resolution once the offending substance is identified.

While this is a separate issue from the substances listed above that are considered toxins, allergens in personal care products deserve mention because they are so common and costly in terms of economic burden to the 14 million Americans each year diagnosed with allergic contact dermatitis.

Identification of the offending substance (which does not have to be a chemical and, in fact, can easily be a natural substance such as an herb) and then strict avoidance of that substance is the cure for this problem. A thorough medical history and patch testing usually yields the identification of the responsible culprit.

Each year, the American Contact Dermatitis Society designates one allergen as Allergen of the Year with the intention of bringing public awareness to it. It is easy to think of airborne allergens and food allergies as causing problems in our bodies, but realizing that substances that we come into active contact with can cause a local allergic reaction is important too. As mentioned above, fragrance won the 2007 Allergen of the Year Award.

While fragrances consist of natural and synthetic ingredients, over 90% of them are synthetic. Fragrances are found in many products such as perfumes, colognes, body sprays, cosmetics, skin-care products, foods, cleaning products, and home air fresheners.

Fragrances have been found to account for 30-45% of allergic contact dermatitis to cosmetics! Fragrances in toothpastes and mouthwashes, chewing gum, and flavored cigarettes may be the cause of oral and perioral dermatitis—a red rash around the mouth.

In 2008, the common metal, nickel, won the award and currently holds the record as the most popular allergen with a prevalence rate of 17% of all people patch tested worldwide. Nickel has traditionally been found in zippers, safety pins, doorknobs, keys, scissors, eyelash curlers, belt buckles, razors, tools, appliances, jewelry, and paper clips.

Currently, nickel-containing electronics, such as cell phones, laptops, iPhones, and iPads have been associated with a systemized nickel reaction. This is an area previously not considered in thinking about nickel sensitivity, but certainly bears consideration today.

Jumping ahead to 2012 we saw acrylates in the hot seat for allergic contact dermatitis. In one study of 257 beauticians identified between 1996 and 2011, acrylates from artificial nails were the most common cause.

I am seeing more of a preservative called methylisothiazolinone in product labels these days. From 2007 to 2010, twice as many U.S. cosmetic products contained methylisothiazolinone and the skyrocketing rates of it causing allergic contact dermatitis earned it the 2013 Allergen of the Year. It is found in bubble solution, bubble baths, soaps, and cosmetic products.

Next, we arrive at the 2015 Allergen of the Year Award, which goes to formaldehyde, an inexpensive and effective preservative. Formaldehyde-releasing systems (see above) are among the leading contact allergens found in personal-care products such as shampoos, body washes, hand soaps, lotions and creams, baby wipes, mascara, disinfectants, fabric softeners, and adhesives. According to the FDA Voluntary Cosmetic Registration Program database, about 20% of personal-care products and cosmetics contain a formaldehyde-releaser system, with imidazolidinyl urea as the most common form of it. Remember, when it comes to formaldehyde-releasing preservative systems, you will not see formaldehyde listed on the label. That's because the chemical ingredient that breaks down into formaldehyde goes by a different name. See the different name of ingredients that are used in formaldehyde-releasing preservative systems in the paragraph on formaldehyde above.

Safer Cosmetics

There exists a very large database that evaluates cosmetics and skin-care products for toxicity concerns and then rates them. It is called the EWG's Skin Deep database and can be found at www.ewg.org. Environmental Working Group (EWG) has 80,000 products in their database and it can be used to evaluate both your current products and products that you are considering.

Another website, www.madesafe.org, screens products' ingredients for the following:

- Behavioral toxins
- Carcinogens
- Developmental toxins
- Endocrine disruptors
- Fire retardants
- GMOs (Genetically Modified Organisms)

- Heavy metals
- Neurotoxins
- Pesticides/insecticides/herbicides
- Reproductive toxins
- Toxic solvents
- VOCs

MadeSafe.org awards two different seals: one for products that have passed the standards listed above, called "Made Safe," and then another label for products that have actually gone through laboratory testing and were found to be non-toxic. This label is the "Non-toxic Certified" label and crosses many consumer categories to give consumers confidence in more than just personal-care products.

Amy Ziff, the founder and executive director of MadeSafe.org recently presented her TED talk titled "It's time to end the creation of toxic soup." This is a must-watch video that may shock you, as the toxic soup that we live in is not even on the radar of conventional medicine.

https://www.youtube.com/watch?v=hX_cF3gSERY

Another option for those on the go is an app called "Think Dirty," which can be downloaded onto your smart phone or other device. This application scans the bar code on the products you already own, and then produces a score based on how the ingredients rated in terms of safety. The "Dirty Meter" looks at carcinogenicity, developmental and reproductive toxicity, allergies, and immunotoxicities. You can also input the name of a product and see how it scores. This app is great to take into a store and scan potential products you may wish to buy to see how the product's ingredients stack up. Once the product is scanned and scored, all the ingredients are listed and scored separately so that you can educate yourself on why a particular ingredient scored poorly.

A drawback to these databases is that the ratings may be based on limited information. Also, the studies that have been done have been done one chemical at a time.

The rising cancer rates should have us questioning many things. For example, what if none of the chemicals tested is carcinogenic (because they are all used in formulations at low doses under the "dose makes the poison" argument), but nearly half of us get cancer? Shouldn't we be more concerned? Perhaps we should be looking at combinations of chemicals? Longer time frames of exposure? As substances applied to skin bypass the first pass liver detoxification system and can be absorbed directly into the bloodstream, the need for extensive and broadly based safety profiles are necessary. Key endpoints to consider in these assessments should include genotoxicity and carcinogenicity, endocrine disruption, and neurotoxicity

Also, an individual may have a skin sensitizing or allergic reaction to an ingredient that has nothing to do with that ingredient's safety profile. There is no way to predict this potential reaction, and botanical or "natural" ingredients are just as prone, or even more likely, to cause a sensitizing reaction as a synthetic ingredient. When choosing what products to use, keep this in mind since allergies are very individual.

Conclusion

Unlike the relatively known concept that whole fresh foods, vegetables, and fruits are healthy, it is hard for anyone to know if a favorite shampoo or lipstick contributes to cancer risk or the health of unborn children. Naturopathic physicians, guided by *prevenir* (to prevent), *docere* (to teach), and *tolle causum* (find the cause), are natural leaders to promote awareness to patients and our greater communities in choosing healthy personal-care and cosmetic products. Reading labels may be our greatest tool in this endeavor.

So what kinds of personal-care products should you use? It is essential to read labels on your personal-care products to know what is really in your bottle. Don't just look at the name of the product. It is perfectly legal right now to call a product Organic Plant Shampoo and then not have any organic ingredients listed on the label, or even in the product for that matter. Of course, that shampoo bottle will also be missing an organic certification seal, such as USDA Organic, because it does not meet the requirements.

After making sure the label does not contain suspect ingredients (discussed in this chapter), look for an organic certification seal. In the U.S., we have the USDA Organic seal, which is green. This seal specifies that 95% of the ingredients are organically sourced. However, you can have a clean personal-care product that is not necessarily certified organic.

Here is an example of a clean personal-care product swap. Most women use a body lotion all over their body after a shower to lock in the moisture content. An easy substitute from the commercially available varieties of body lotion (all filled with petroleum products, parabens, and other questionable ingredients) is plain coconut oil. That's right. Buy a good quality coconut oil suitable for cooking and put it in your bathroom. After toweling off, apply to your body just like you would a commercial body lotion. Don't be put off by the fact that it will be liquid in the summer and hardened in the winter. If it is hard, it will quickly melt into your hands and onto your body. Because there is no alcohol in coconut oil, it will not dry quickly on your skin. For this reason, wait a few minutes for it to sink into your skin and towel off the excess so that you can get dressed. If you don't have anywhere to go right away, take your time in having your skin soak up this healing oil.

Applying the information

The Minimalist

- Go fragrance free. Throw out the plug-in, synthetic air fresheners, scented candles, perfume, cologne, and laundry detergent, and start buying only scent-free or non-fragranced skin-care products.

The Middle Way: Accompanying the above,

- Change out your underarm deodorant to a paraben- and aluminum-free version.

The Beauty Buff: In Addition to All of the above,

- Review all of your cosmetic and skin-care products, read labels, run products through the Think Dirty app, consult with EWG.org, or look for certified products on MadeSafe.org and choose the healthiest replacements that you can.

Nutritional Strategies for All 21 Days

ARE YOU READY FOR A BEAUTY TRANSFORMATION? It's time to put into practice what this book talks about and use the power of nutrition, stress reduction, beauty sleep, targeted supplements, and cleaner personal care products to fuel and reveal your true radiance.

Begin by establishing an anti-inflammatory diet which will nourish your skin and flood your body with antioxidants.

Top Inflammatory Foods to Avoid

- Sugar
- Alcohol
- Feedlot raised meats
- Dairy products
- Common cooking oils like cottonseed, sunflower, safflower
- Transfat
- Refined grains

- Any food to which you are sensitive

To eat for beauty is to be mindful of consuming an organic, anti-inflammatory diet, which is rich in whole foods, vegetables and fruits, legumes with plenty of healthy fats (rather than processed vegetable oils), and avoiding processed foods, even if they are labeled gluten free or organic. I advise eating real food!

Eliminate the following foods from your diet completely:

- Wheat and other gluten-containing grains (e.g. rye, barley, and oats1)
- Dairy
- Eggs
- Corn
- Soy
- Peanuts
- Sugar
- Alcohol

The first seven items on this list are the top allergenic foods, which lead to inflammation, a leading contributor to poor skin health and wrinkles. By removing these foods, you will not only reveal more youthful skin, but you will probably also *shed pounds, gain energy, and increase mental clarity.*

The average American now eats 22 teaspoons of sugar per day. This is truly terrible for both our health and our complexion. While

---

[1] While oats are naturally gluten-free, most commercial oats are processed in factories where wheat is also present, and cross-contamination is common, so avoid oats unless they are specifically labeled as gluten-free.

removing sugar from your diet sounds extremely difficult to do, you will find that after just three days of avoiding sugar, while at the same time increasing healthy fats, you will lose your craving for sugar and feel better than ever (although for some people with blood-sugar issues, this may take longer).

A good tip to get through those days is to make sure to have plenty of good unsalted raw nuts around to snack on, such as walnuts, almonds, or macadamia nuts, or nut butters which are naturally rich in protein and fat.

Also, watch out for common sources of hidden sugar, including protein bars, protein drinks, all processed foods, sodas, fruit juices, baked goods, and coffee drinks.

Alcohol is an inflammatory drink and also changes your gut microbiome, which in turn affects your skin negatively, so remove it from your diet for this period and watch your skin transform.

Feed your skin these antioxidant-rich foods (ensuring you always choose organic, of course):

- Apples
- Asparagus
- Avocado
- Beets
- Blackberries, blueberries, raspberries, strawberries
- Cherries
- Broccoli
- Chocolate/cocoa
- Ginger

- Green tea
- Kale, spinach, and other dark leafy greens
- Olive oil
- Parsley
- Pears
- Plums
- Pomegranate

In addition, choose from the following foods that activate your Nrf-2 molecule, which produces internal antioxidants and detoxifying enzymes (and again, whichever you choose, make sure they are organic).

Foods and spices that activate Nrf-2:

- Green tea
- Broccoli and other cruciferous vegetables
- Ginger
- Garlic
- Curcumin
- Olive oil
- Fish oil
- Lycopene (tomatoes, red/pink grapefruit, watermelon, papaya, mango)

While no one diet will work for everyone, these foods are the cornerstone for healthy and nourishing nutrition:

- Organic, grass-fed, pasture-raised meats and wild-caught fish
- Organic vegetables (non-starchy)
- Organic potatoes and other roots (starchy)

- Organic nuts & seeds (walnut, pumpkin, chia, flax, hemp)
- Organic fruits (berries are awesome, especially wild blueberries)
- Organic fermented foods (sauerkraut, kim chi, miso)
- Organic healthy fats (grass-fed butter or ghee, coconut oil, avocados)

Days 1 to 3 - How to Detox your Diet: The Sugar Detox

Go cold turkey. It's the only way you will be able to get off the sugar treadmill. You know what I'm talking about: that continual searching for sugar all day long, which starts to feel inescapable after a while. Eventually, you get to the point where you don't believe you can function or think without sugar. The resulting seesaw creates an imbalance in your blood sugar, and you swing from feeling good to feeling bad, irritable, and downright cranky. Eliminating sugar makes for stable moods, improved energy, and increased productivity.

For these first three days, crank up the good fats. When you are preparing your morning smoothie, add coconut oil, Medium Chain Triglycerides (MCT) oil—which is derived from coconut—or Omega-3 essential fatty acids, such as fish oil. Be sure to eat nuts, especially walnuts for their Omega-3 essential fatty acid content, and add almond butter to your morning smoothie as well. Our brains are predominantly comprised of fat, and most people perform better cognitively when they have abundant healthy fats in their diets. The low-fat craze of the 70s and 80s turned out tor be a nutritional disaster as the fat-free alternatives simply substituted sugar to perk up the flavor once the tastiness of the fat was removed.

> **Sample Smoothie:**
> - 1 cup organic almond milk (or ~~can go~~ half water and half almond milk)
> - 2 scoops protein powder (pea or rice)
> - 1 tablespoon virgin coconut oil
> - ½ cup of organic blueberries or strawberries (optional)
> - 1 teaspoon almond or cashew butter
> - 1 tablespoon tocotrienols
> - 1 teaspoon MSM powder
> - 1/2 teaspoon camu camu powder or other vitamin C powder

NOTE: Tocotrienols, MSM powder and camu camu powder are supplements that are good for the skin, however MSM powder and camu camu powder can throw off the taste of your smoothie. One way to get around that is to pour most of your shake into your glass, then add the MSM and camu camu powder to what is left in the blender, blend, pour this into a separate glass and drink it first. Then you can enjoy the rest of your delicious shake. Alternatively, leave out the MSM and camu camu.

If you don't drink smoothies for breakfast, a convenient way to get your healthy fats, protein, and fiber is to mix together a delicious blend of chia seeds, buckwheat groats, dried cranberries or fresh berries, shelled hemp seeds, and chopped walnuts in a bowl and soak them in almond milk for 15 minutes.

Chia puddings are another great breakfast that is rich in healthy fats and fiber, and the Internet is full of delicious recipes for them. Find one that can be made the night before, and you'll have a quick and easy breakfast in the morning.

If you are having freshly prepared vegetable juice, I recommend adding a little olive oil and staying away from large quantities of sweet produce such as carrots, beets, apples, and other fruits. I have seen a lot of *juice cleanses* on the market that contain astronomical amounts of sugar!

Dr. Fine's Skin Beauty Juice Recipe

For best results use organic fruits and vegetables; if not, you are just putting concentrated pesticides into a glass and drinking them.

- 1 carrot (optional for those with sugar issues)
- 4 stalks of celery
- 1 large handful parsley
- 1 large handful spinach
- ¼ beet
- 1-2 inches of ginger (can work your way up)
- 1-2 cloves of garlic (occasionally, not every day)
- 1/3 to 1/2 cucumber
- ½ lemon

If you are simply practical, go ahead and eat your leftovers from the night before which hopefully contain protein, fats, and vegetables. There is no rule that says you have to stick to "breakfast" foods. Wild salmon for breakfast, anyone?

What's not on the breakfast menu? Cereal, toast, bagels, fruit juice: these items are way too sugary and unsatisfying to start your day properly. While you may protest that a bagel isn't inherently sweet, the refined grains in it simply turn to sugar in your bloodstream. This applies to gluten-free foods as well, which are still processed grains, low in fiber, and refined.

For mid-morning snacks, I would suggest raw nuts, a protein powder drink (without added sugar; some use stevia or lucuma, or xylitol), some hummus and raw vegetables.

For lunch and dinner, continue with robust and clean sources of proteins, healthy fats, and organic vegetables. Be mindful of making your meals both flavorsome and full of fiber. That way, they will fill you up and satisfy your taste buds, and you won't feel the need for sweets after meals.

If you eat animal products, be sure to buy grass-fed beef, free-range chickens, and wild salmon or other fish that are low in mercury.

If you simply must have a sweet treat, I recommend keeping some organic Medjool dates in the freezer and having *one*! They taste even more decadent when they are frozen.

Also, dark chocolate is on the "yes!" list due to its high percentage of flavanols. Look for 65% or higher chocolate: the higher the dark chocolate content, the lower the sugar. Limit yourself to one square per day, and preferably choose organic. If you find this just increases your sugar cravings, then go without chocolate, at least for the duration of this 21-day period.

Days 4 to 6 - How to Detox your Beauty Routine

Over the next three days you are going to go through your personal-care products and makeup to see what's really in them. Then you will prepare to eliminate them from your life and start choosing cleaner options.

I realize not everyone will have the budget and the time to make a clean sweep right away, but do the detective work now, and start strategically purging your products as they run out by replacing them with better products.

One quick way to get started is to load the free app Think Dirty on your smartphone, go into your bathroom, and start scanning your beauty products to see how they rate. You can also go to www.ewg.org to check specific products. This makes it so much easier!

As a doctor who focuses on environmental medicine, I was shocked when I finally began investigating the personal-care product industry, and how the ingredients it uses are contributing to our overall body burden of chemicals and causing us to feel sick and tired.

There is no getting around the fact that you must go through your entire beauty routine, throwing out the toxic products, and replacing them with clean alternatives. In addition, you must learn how to read the labels, as relying on words like "natural" or "organic" or "non-toxic" on the label may be misleading. Here is the general list of ingredients that are best avoided, and the names by which they are often listed on the label:

- Phthalates:
    - Fragrance
    - Parfum

- Parabens:
    - Methylparaben,
    - Propylparaben,
    - Butylparaben,

- o Ethylparaben
- o Iso-Butylparaben
- Triclosan or triclocarban

- Ethoxylated ingredients that can be contaminated with 1-4 dioxane (a carcinogen):
  - o Sodium laureth sulfate
  - o Polyethylene
  - o Polyethylene glycol (PEG)
  - o Polyoxyethylene
  - o Polysorbate
  - o Or any ingredient with "-xynol", "ceteareth", or "oleth"
- Formaldehyde releasers:
  - o quaternium-15
  - o dimethyl-dimethyl (DMDM) hydantoin
  - o imidazolidinyl urea
  - o diazolidinyl urea
  - o 2-bromo-2-nitropropane-1,3-diol (bronopol)
  - o sodium hydroxymethylglycinate
- Amines:
  - o Triethanolamine or TEA
  - o Diethanolamine or DEA
  - o Monoethanolamine or MEA
- Petrolatum
- Fragrance or "parfum"

DAY 4

Replace:

- Deodorant
- Sunscreen

Your deodorant normally contains xenoestrogens (phthalates and parabens) and metalloestrogens (aluminum), so consider switching to a DIY deodorant such as baking soda. The most basic alternative: after showering and towel drying, simply shake a little baking soda into your palm and gently press it into the opposite underarm. Switch hands and repeat for the other underarm. Afterwards, lightly brush off any excess baking soda with your hands, and wash your hands so that you don't drop powder on your clothes.

Baking soda is a natural, safe and inexpensive defense against odor. For many of you who don't sweat much, or live in cooler climates, this may be all you need.

For others, an alternative is to purchase a clean deodorant, but beware of greenwashing: this is a marketing technique used to mislead consumers into believing that a product is "green" or non-toxic by using unregulated terms such as "natural" on the label. A prime example of greenwashing is the case of a well-known and trusted manufacturer of baking soda that developed a "natural" deodorant which proudly proclaimed on the front label, "no parabens or aluminum." Closer examination of the ingredients, however, revealed that the product contained Triclosan, an antibacterial agent and suspected endocrine disruptor. This deception resulted in a class action lawsuit which was eventually settled.

Fortunately, there are many authentic non-toxic deodorants on the market. You can check products using the Think Dirty app, or search for them in the Skin Deep database on www.ewg.org, or on www.madesafe.org.

Your second step is to rid yourself of the most toxic product in your skin care routine, sunscreen. Commercial sunscreens are some of the most toxic products available; in addition to the usual suspects of questionable ingredients such as parabens and phthalates, they also contain chemical UV filters such as oxybenzone. The CDC reports that oxybenzone was found in nearly all Americans tested in their ongoing body burden program.

Most chemical sunscreens use one or more chemicals that are suspected endocrine disruptors and work by chemically reacting with the skin to avoid sun and DNA damage. Physical sunscreens, on the other hand, contain active minerals such as zinc oxide and titanium oxide, and simply sit on top of the skin and deflect the UV rays. So, replace your chemical sunscreen with a physical sunscreen that contains zinc oxide, or a combination of zinc oxide and titanium oxide, and preferably also contains antioxidants.

DAY 5

Replace:

- Shampoo and Conditioner
- Liquid soaps
- Shaving creams
- Body lotion
- Facial moisturizers, including anti-aging products

Foaming and sudsing cleansers such as shampoos and body washes are filled with questionable ingredients. Natural alternatives often do not foam as much, but the amount of suds or foam produced does not determine whether a product is an effective cleanser.

I have always been a fan of Dr. Bronner's Pure-Castile liquid soaps, which have been on the market for decades and are as pure as they come. Many newer, non-toxic, liquid soaps have also entered the marketplace, so it should be easy to replace what you already have. Remember, if Triclosan is listed as an ingredient, do not purchase that product.

A shaving tip for both men and women is to forego the shaving cream, as it contains many ingredients that should be avoided. As a natural alternative, smooth jojoba oil on your skin just prior to shaving. (Yes, ladies, you can do this in the shower.) The beauty of using jojoba or similar oils is that they work like shaving cream, and the razor glides over the slicked skin. As an added bonus, your skin will retain some of that hydration after you get out of the shower.

Where body lotions are concerned, I recommend coconut oil. I keep one jar for use in the kitchen, and another jar in the bathroom to apply after a shower. Coconut oil is a pure and natural product; it does not contain alcohol, fragrances (which include phthalates), parabens, synthetic silicones, and other ingredients that you find in mass-produced body lotions. However, since coconut oil doesn't contain alcohol, you must wait a few minutes for it to absorb into your skin, or it will get on your clothing. In more humid climates, you may need to blot off the excess.

Facial creams, especially the anti-aging creams, contain toxic ingredients that actually produce inflammation in your skin, which will lead to even faster aging! Indeed, it was the toxic ingredients in anti-aging creams that inspired me to formulate my own non-toxic, anti-aging oil-based serum. Today, safer and more effective anti-aging creams and oil-based serums are being introduced and changing what's possible in creating and maintaining natural beauty and radiance in your skin.

For a luxurious and pampering experience on your skin try a European face oil. The formulation of my own IAMFINE Youth Serum was based on my training in Europe. I have traveled the globe to carefully source all the superior ingredients found in my products, and I only use the highest quality plant materials. My products do not contain cheap, low-grade filler oils. By using only, the highest quality ingredients my Eco-Luxury brand is effective at skin transformation.

DAY 6

Replace

- Perfumes, colognes
- Foundation
- Lipstick
- Mascara
- Eyeliner and eye makeup

"Fragrance" is a catch-all term used by manufacturers to disguise phtalates and other "trade secret" ingredients that are known to be endocrine disruptors and skin sensitizers. Often, when people have a reaction to products on their skin, they are actually reacting to the fragrance. Eliminating fragrance or scents in personal care products often makes a dramatic difference in how you will feel. The same applies to the cleaning products you use around the house, such as scented laundry detergent and dryer sheets. So, replace the perfumes, colognes, and other fragranced products in your current beauty programs. And remember: *nearly all products contain fragrance.*

If you are someone who has a reaction going down the laundry aisle in the grocery store, you may be chemically sensitive and be reacting to the fragrances.

Decades before I became aware of these toxins, this was me. Intuitively, I began avoiding all fragrances, including the perfume that I thought every woman must apply before leaving the house to be "properly dressed." I couldn't imagine not wearing my signature scent. Even so, I discarded it, and I asked my husband to abandon his cologne as well. In addition, we started buying unscented products for the home. I felt much better as a result, although at the time I didn't really understand why.

As well as fragrances, makeup is often contaminated with heavy metals. Although rare, mercury is sometimes used as a preservative for mascara, and many lipsticks, especially red, contain lead.

Of course, it's one thing knowing what to avoid. But what should you use instead? Armed with the above list of chemicals, go to your nearest health-food store and browse their selection of personal-care products. Alternatively, visit sites such as The Detox Market, which is a curated site for natural and organic skin care and personal care products. You will find better choices there and a wide variety of products, ranging from baby-care to anti-aging, and even men's care. In addition, use the resources mentioned in the previous section: www.madesafe.org lists safe products, the Think Dirty app allows you to to check potential new beauty products in-store using your smartphone, and you can consult with www.ewg.org for their Skin Deep database ratings. Please note that none of these product or ingredient ratings is perfect, but they are a good starting guide.

Days 7 to 10 - How to Detox Stress from Your Life

Now that you are detoxifying on the physical level, it is time to work on the emotional level and address the stress in your life. Remember, stress stimulates the production of cortisol, which causes premature aging of the skin by breaking down collagen and elastin, and promotes dryness and redness in the skin. Excess cortisol also makes it difficult to get your beauty sleep.

DAY 7

Being more organized is a stress-reliever. Being on time to work and to meetings is a stress-reliever. Arriving at the airport early is a stress-reliever. Don't underestimate the stress-relieving effect of simply being where you need to be a few minutes early.

Lay out your work clothes in the evening, before you go to bed. That way, when you get up in the morning you have one less thing to stress over, and you're not trying to match outfits while rushing to get out of the house.

In the morning, set your alarm a few minutes earlier than you normally would and give yourself those few minutes to mentally and emotionally prepare for your day.

How you start your day sets the tone for the rest of the day, so cultivate a habit of being grateful. Start with a five minute gratitude period when you wake. This can be done in bed. Give thanks for everything you can think of for which you are grateful, including the ability to be able to get out of bed: Not everyone can get out of bed in the morning. For bonus points, start a gratitude journal, and write down the list of things you are grateful for each day.

DAY 8

Incorporate "earthing" into your day. Find a patch of grass, sandy beach, or other natural ground, remove your shoes and just come in contact with the earth in your bare feet. If you can, take a walk, but if you are in your backyard, just do some yardwork or gardening, or simpy relax there. Take stock of how you feel before you start this exercise and after. In particular, if you have any pain, rate it on a scale of 1 to 10 with 10 being the highest pain, before and after.

DAY 9

Get thee into nature today. Do some "forest bathing." If you are fortunate enough to live near a forest, take the opportunity to walk in the woods as often as you like. If you don't live near woods, but you find yourself near one—say on vacation or while traveling—make time to take a walk in it.

Being out in any green area is calming, however, so the next best thing is to get out into a park or an area with greenery, even if it is entirely surrounded by high-rise buildings: Central Park, is a prime example.

And finally, if all you can manage is to look out your window at some greenery, this too has been proven to reduce stress, improve attention—even in children with ADHD—increase longevity, reduce blood pressure, and improve mood.

DAY 10

Today is the day to add in an on-the-spot stress buster. Experiment with the following options to find one that can be your go-to stress reset button:

- At a really stressful point, stop and take three deep breaths. This will serve to calm you down instantly, and even temporarily lower blood pressure.
- Essential oils used for aromatherapy are a great tool to ease your stress, and the bottles are tiny and fit easily into your purse. Inhaling lavender provides an immediate calming response, as do vetiver, chamomile, and frankincense.
- It is natural to want to avoid strong emotions, because we don't like the physical feelings they create. Recognizing that our emotions are only temporary is a wonderful insight that will stand you in good stead. Understand that the physical sensations of the unpleasant emotion you are experiencing

will normally not last more than a couple of minutes, and just breathe. This is very powerful.

- If your body hangs on to the stress response, then a physical activity, such as a long walk, yoga, swimming, a workout with weights, or tai chi as soon as you can get to it—even if you have to wait until evening—will dissipate the surge in cortisol.

Days 11 to 14 - How to Incorporate Targeted Supplements for a Beauty Boost

The nutricosmetics market—consumable nutritional supplements designed to provide hydration, nourishment, antioxidant activity, and other beauty benefits to improve the appearance of skin, hair, and nails from the inside out—is expected to reach $7.4 billion in the US by 2020, according to Global Industry Analysts (GIA).

This trend was slow to gain traction in the United States, but the US is now the fastest growing market for nutricosmetics. There are so many supplements and nutricosmetics to choose from that it's difficult to choose, so here are my top picks.

Basic supplements that are foundational for good skin health:

- Vitamin C (from non-corn sources)
- B Complex (with methylated folic acid and B12)
- Vitamin D (consult a medical professional and arrange a blood test to ensure you take the correct dose for you)
- Zinc

- Vitamin E – tocotrienols and tocopherols
- Probiotics (consult a naturopathic doctor and get a professional brand and based on your microbiome)
- Selenium

A high quality multivitamin should contain most, if not all, of these nutrients with the exception of probiotics. If you are taking one of these high-quality multivitamins, there is no added benefit from taking additional supplements of the same vitamins (e.g. a separate Vitamin E supplement): all you will be doing is exceeding the recommended daily amount. In this case, more is not better.

Disclaimer: It is always best to consult with your naturopathic doctor as to the recommended dosages and supplements that are right for you, as your doctor can assess you and perform laboratory testing to check your levels.

DAY 11

Review your current supplements to see if your high-quality multivitamin contains the vitamins and minerals listed above. In addition, it is advisable to have your nutrient status properly assessed by a naturopathic doctor. The results will guide you in choosing the appropriate supplementation for your metabolism.

The supplements available at big box stores are often full of fillers and cheap, poorly absorbed, and often inactive versions of the vitamins and minerals. Through your naturopathic doctor you will have also access to professional lines of supplements produced by pharmaceutical companies who adhere to strict industry and pharmaceutical standards.

DAY 12

Add astaxanthin to your regimen, and fish oil, if you are not already taking it.

DAY 13

Add grape seed extract to your regimen.

DAY 14

If you are not eating bone broth, increase your collagen intake by adding a collagen powder or ingestible (see Resources) to your diet.

Days 15 to 18 - How to Get Your Beauty Sleep

There is no beauty without beauty sleep!

A single night of lost sleep has been shown to epigenetically alter the genes that control the biological clocks in cells throughout the body, accelerating aging, so getting a good night's sleep is critical to your skincare regimen.

DAY 15

Quick Start Sleep Protocol

Aim for 7-8 hours a night. According to Chinese Medicine, the best and most rejuvenating sleep is before midnight, so be in bed by 10:00 pm.

It is possible to retrain your circadian rhythms relatively easily. If you currently go to bed later than 10:00 pm, start to train yourself by going to bed 30 minutes earlier than usual tonight. Then tomorrow night, go to bed another 30 minutes earlier, and so on until you have brought your bedtime forward to 10:00 pm.

Reorganize your day to carve out a one-hour period before bed, then pick two or more actions from the list below, and do them each night for the two-day period.

- Use this hour to do yoga or tai chi. If these activities are new to you, there are many local classes and online courses that will teach you the moves so you can do them on your own later.
- Talk a walk. Walking is underestimated as a stress-relieving activity. Review your day and clear your mind.
- Read a non-work book. Reading before bed is very relaxing, and a book of fiction will allow you to escape your stress, imagine a different world, and engage in someone else's story. Inspirational and spiritual books are also good choices. Read to escape, or read to inspire and uplift.
- Whatever your spiritual frame of reference, tap into your relationship with the Divine, learn to relish the unique talents you have been given. Strategize how best to unleash them upon the world for the greater good and fulfillment of your sacred contract. Be you, in all your glory.
- Writing is very therapeutic, and some find that once they put their thoughts on paper, they no longer have to think about them. If you are anxious about something now or in the future, write it down and put it out of your mind. You can also journal your day to create a more regular writing habit.

- I don't recommend a glass of wine before bed because, while it may facilitate falling asleep, it will often interfere with staying asleep. Instead, enjoy a bedtime beverage such as chamomile tea or another herbal blend.

- Create a relaxing space to end your day. Enjoy a warm bath with Epsom salts and essential oils such as lavender, play soft music, and dim the lights.

Understand that your day is done; it is complete. It is no longer necessary to review or obsess over any of its parts anymore. Your reward, a peaceful slumber, is right around the corner, and you deserve it.

DAY 16

One hour before bed, at 9:00 pm, power down all of your electronics, and then power down yourself:

- Meditation
- Guided meditation (look to the internet for resources)
- Breath work
- Journaling
- Tai chi
- Prayer
- Visualization
- Inspirational reading

If you need more help in getting to sleep, add one or more of the following:

- A cup of chamomile tea

- Melatonin
- Hops tincture

Other considerations:

- Caffeine dissipates more slowly in some individuals and as a result it can keep them awake at night. If caffeine is impinging on your ability to sleep, eliminate caffeinated beverages completely or only have them in the morning.
- Some people find a nighttime workout is too stimulating and will prevent them falling asleep. If that is you, do your workout in the morning
- Your body has evolved to respond to the way daylight changes throughout the day. F.Lux is software for your computer and mobile devices that mimics the natural change at the end of the day by reducing blue light from your screen. This free download can be found at https://justgetflux.com/

DAY 17

Ambient light reduces melatonin, the chemical your brain produces to trigger sleep. Make sure your room is cool and, above all, dark and wear an eye mask to keep out any remaining light. A more permanent, but also more expensive, solution is to invest in blackout shades for your windows, which completely entomb your bedroom in darkness, thus protecting and preserving your precious supply of melatonin.

Keep a clear and safe path to the bathroom. That way, should you need to go in the night, you will not need to turn on the lights. If you do need to keep a night light on, a sleep mask will be even more important.

DAY 18

Restrict fluids before bed and stop eating three hours before bedtime to ensure you can get through the night without waking up, thus allowing the body to rest and repair properly.

Days 19 to 21 - How to Detox your Body

DAY 19

Invest in a skin brush, easily obtained from your local health-food store or over the internet. Start dry brushing your skin in the morning after you wake up. This should take only about five minutes and will jump start your lymph system to dump toxins into your bloodstream for removal.

DAY 20

Support your liver by including the following foods in your diet:

- Beets
- Parsley
- Lemon and lemon juice (you can start the day with ½ lemon in warm water)
- Burdock root (which can be juiced)
- Artichokes
- Leafy greens (Dandelion greens are especially helpful)

- Watercress
- Garlic
- Asparagus
- Apples

For added punch, add juiced, grated or chopped turmeric and ginger to your diet. You can buy turmeric rhizome in health food stores, and ginger root in the produce department of your grocery store.

The absolutely easiest way to incorporate the most liver cleansing foods into your dietary routine is to juice them. Most of the ingredients listed above can be juiced—refer back to the Dr. Fine Beauty Juice recipe above and simply augment your juice with some added liver detoxifiers.

In addition, stay away from the beauty betrayers that clog up your liver and ruin your complexion:

- Alcohol
- Caffeine
- Fried foods including chips of all kinds, even the "healthy" ones
- Sugar
- Vegetable oils (with the exception of extra virgin olive oil)
- Unnecessary over-the-counter drugs like NSAIDS, PPIs (acid inhibitors), and recreational drugs
- Cigarettes

DAY 21

Sweat

- Sauna
- Exercise

Sauna therapy is great for skin and overall body tissue detoxification or tissue cleansing. Ideally, every home would have one which the entire family could use. Alternatively, you will find them in many gyms. I recommend dry sauna as the steam saunas can harbor mold.

As I mentioned earlier, exercise reduces stress. Additionally, it also increases circulation, which is good for your skin.

The End of the Journey, Or Just the Beginning?

Congratulations on stopping the clock—you've done it! You are 21 days into new habits, and you will see a distinct change in your facial skin and tone. Your face will be clear, radiant, depuffed and plumper, and your wrinkles and fine lines will be less noticeable. You will also enjoy greater energy with no more energy crashes during the day, you will sleep better, your brain will function better, you will have lost some weight, and you will feel and look years younger!

By using solutions that address the root of aging, you have slowed, and possibly even reversed, your extrinsic and intrinsic aging processes, both on the inside of your body and the outside. Your skin has been reset into a more virtuous cycle, and going forward, you can enjoy even more youthful-looking skin, better health, and vitality.

Resources

Dr. Anne Marie Fine, N.M.D.
www.drannemariefine.com
Newport Beach, CA
Telephone: 949-650-3333
Email: info@drannemariefine.com

Dr. Fine is available for virtual appointments, on a limited basis. Her website and blog also include a great deal of useful information about natural medicine, environmental medicine, and natural beauty.

Fine Natural Products, LLC
www.iamfineskin.com
Dr. Anne Marie Fine
Founder & C.E.O.
Newport Beach, CA
Telephone: 844-IAMFINE

This is where you can purchase IAMFINE® Pure Skin Collection and also access great articles.

Other IAMFINE® Resources

Facebook:

www.facebook.com/drannemariefine/

Facebook:

www.facebook.com/Dr-Anne-Marie-Fine-314085772261291/

Twitter:

@DrAnneMarieFine

Instagram:

IAMFINEbyDrAnneMarieFine

Digital Class on Clean Beauty:

http://bit.ly/beautybluff

More information on Frequency Specific Microcurrent Device:

http://bit.ly/FSMDev

Naturopathic and Environmental Medicine Doctors

American Association of Naturopathic Physicians:

www.naturopathic.org

Naturopathic Academy of Environmental Medicine: www.naturopathicenvironment.com

Online Education for Environmental Medicine:

Progressive Medical Education

An online member organization committed to the latest research and education in Environmental Medicine and it's impact on our personal health.

www.progressivemedicaleducation.com

Personal Care Product Ingredient Safety

Environmental Working Group: www.ewg.org

Made Safe: www.madesafe.org

Think Dirty app: www.thinkdirtyapp.com

Beauty Food

Dr. Amy Bader and her team at Real Beauty Food, Inc. formulated real beauty foods featuring skin beautifying herbs and collagen that help create and maintain beautiful skin. Their product line called SkinTē® can be purchased in a glass bottle (no BPA) and the low sugar dessert products eaten as is.

www.realbeautyfood.com

References

Chapter 1

Brooks-Wilson A. Genetics of healthy aging and longevity. *Hum Genet.* 2013; 132(12): 1323–1338.

Slieker R. et al. Age-related accrual of methylomic variability is linked to fundamental ageing mechanisms *Genome Biology* 2016 17:191.

Anand P. et al. Cancer is a preventable disease that requires major lifestyle changes. *Pharm Res* 2008;25(9):2097-2116.

Hughes MCB, et al. Sunscreen and Prevention of Skin Aging. *Ann Intern Med.* 2013;158:I-28.

Khan SI et al. Epigenetic events associated with breast cancer and their prevention by dietary components targeting the epigenome. *Chem Res Toxicol* 2012 Jan 13:25(1):61-73.

Ong TP et al. Targeting the epigenome with bioactive food components for cancer prevention. *J Nutrigenet Nutrigenomics* 2012 Feb;4(5):275-292.

Vierkotter, A, Krutmann J. Environmental influences on skin aging and ethnic specific manifestations. *Dermatoendocrinol.* 2012;4(3): 227-31.

Rinnethaler M, et al. Oxidative stress in aging human skin. *Biomolecules* 2015 Apr 21;5(2):545-89.

Thornfeldt C. Viewpoint: Anti-inflammation and visible skin aging. *Skin Inc* 2008 Apr

(http://www.cdc.gov/chronicdisease/ accessed 6/30/12)

Baumann L. Skin ageing and its treatment. *J Pathol* 2007 Jan;211(2):241-51.

Sandovici I. et al. "Maternal Diet and Aging Alter the Epigenetic Control of a Promoter-

Enhancer Interaction at the Hnf4A Gene in Rat Pancreatic Iislets." *Proc Natl Acad Sci USA* 108/13 (2011):5449-54.

Epstein H. Will epigenetics change our approach to treating skin conditions. Skinmed 2013 Nov-Dec;11(6):362-363.

Perner D, Vierkotter A, Surgiri D, et al. Association between sun-exposure, smoking behavior, and serum antioxidant levels with the different manifestations of skin aging signs between Japanese and German women- a pilot study. *J Dermato Sci* 2011;62;138-40.

Raymond Noordam, et al., "High serum glucose levels are associated with a higher perceived age," AGE, February 2013; 35(1):189-195

Jeanmaire C, et al. Glycation during human dermal intrinsic and actinic ageing: an in vivo and in vitro model study. *Br J Dermatol* 2001 Jul;145(1):10-18.

Ozdemir O. et al. Preventative and therapeutic probiotic use in allergic skin condition: experimental and clinical findings. *Biomed Res Int* 2013:Sept 1: doi:10.1155/2013/932391.

Hawrelak J. et al. The causes of intestinal dysbiosis: a review. Alt Med Rev 2004:9(2):180-197.

Humbert P. et al. Intestinal permeability in patients with psoriasis. *J Dermatol Sci* 1991 Jul;2(4):324-326.

Muizzudin N. et al. Physiological effect of probiotic on skin. *J Cosmet Sci* 2012 Nov-Dec;63(6):385-395.

Jackson P. et al. Intestinal permeability in patients with eczema and food allergy. *Lancet* 1981 Jan 13;1(8233):1285-1286.

Hardy H. et al. Probiotics, prebiotics and immunomodulation of gut mucosal defenses: homeostasis and immunopathology. *Nutrients* 2013 June;5(6):1869-1912.

Khalif I. et al. Alterations in the colonic flora and intestinal permeability and evidence of immune activation in chronic constipation. *Dig Liver Dis* 2005 Nov;37(11):838-49.

Hegazy S. et al. Effect of probiotics on pro-inflammatory cytokines and NF-kappaB activation in ulcerative colitis. *World J Gastroenterol* 2010 Sept 7;16(33):4145-51.

http://www.medscape.com/viewarticle/551998 accessed 10/27/15

Madser K. Enhancement of epithelial barrier function by probiotics. *J Epith Bio and Pharm* 2012;5(Suppl-M8):55-59.

Shen Qi et al. Epidermal Stem Cells and Their Epigenetic Regulation Int J Mol Sci. 2013 Sep; 14(9): 17861–17880.

Chapter 2

Choi SW et al. Epigenetics: A new bridge between nutrition and health. *Adv Nutr* 2010 Nov;1(1):8-16.

Crews D et al. Epigenetics transgenerational inheritance of altered stress responses. *Proc Natl Acad Sci USA* 2012 Jun 5;109(23):9143-8.

Genuis SJ. What's out there making us sick? *J of Environ Public Health* 2012;2012:605137.

(http://www.cdc.gov/chronicdisease/ accessed 6/30/12)

S.H. Reuben for the President's Cancer Panel, US Department of Health and Human Services, National Institutes of Health, National Cancer Institute. Reducing Environmental Cancer Risk. What We Can Do Now, 2010, http://deainfo.nci.nih.gov/advisory/pcp/annualReports/pcp08-09rpt/PCP_Report_08-09_508.pdf.

Sears, ME and Genuis SJ, "Environmental Determinants of Chronic Disease and Medical Approaches: Recognition, Avoidance, Supportive

Therapy, and Detoxification," Journal of Environmental and Public Health, vol. 2012, Article ID 356798, 15 pages, 2012. doi:10.1155/2012/356798

Gluckman PD et al. Towards a new developmental synthesis: adaptive developmental plasticity and human disease. *Lancet* 2009 May 9;373(9675):1654-7.

Gronniger E et al. Aging and chronic sun exposures cause distinct epigenetic changes in human skin. *PLoS Genet* 2010 May 27;6(5):e1000971.

Holliday R. Epigenetics: A historical overview. *Epigenetics* 2006 Apr-Jun; 1(2):76-80.

Jirtle RL and Skinner MK. Environmental epigenomics and disease susceptibility. *Nat Rev Genet* 2007 Apr;8(4):253-62.

Katigar SK et al. Epigenetic alterations in ultraviolet radiation-induce skin carcinogenesis: interactions of bioactive dietary components on epigenetic targets. *Phytochem Photobiol* 2012 Sep-Oct;88(5): 1066-74.

Kim KY et al. Association of low-dose exposure to persistent organic pollutants with global DNA hypomethylation in healthy Koreans. *Environ Health Perspect* 2010 Mar;118(3);370-4.

Khan SI et al. Epigenetic events associated with breast cancer and their prevention by dietary components targeting the epigenome. *Chem Res Toxicol* 2012 Jan13;25(1):61-73.

Meaney MJ et al. Epigenetic mechanisms of perinatal programming of hypothalamic-pituitary-adrenal function and health. *Trends Mol Med* 2007 Jul;13(7):269-77.

Meeran S et al. Epigenetic targets of bioactive dietary components for cancer prevention and therapy. *Clin Epigenetics* 2010 Dec;1(3-4):101-116.

http://www8.nationalacademies.org/onpinews/newsitem.aspx?RecordID=10490. Accessed 10/18/15

Papoutisis AJ et al. Resveratrol prevents epigenetic silencing of BRCA-1 by the aromatic hydrocarbon receptor in human breast cancer cells. *J Nutr* 2010 September 140(9):1607-1614.

Pereira F et al. Vitamin D has wide regulatory effects on histone demethylase genes. Cell Cycle 2012 Mar 15;11(6):1081-9.

Su LI et al. Epigenetic contributions to the relationship between cancer and dietary intake of nutrients, bioactive food components, and environmental toxicants. *Front Genet* 201;2:91.

Slomko H et al. Minireview: Epigenetics of obesity and diabetes in humans. *Endocrinology* 2012 Mar:153(3):1025-30.

Thayer ZM et al. Biological memories of past environments. *Epigenetics* July 2011;6:7:1-6.

Ziesel, S.H. Epigenetic Mechanisms for Nutritional Determinants of Later Health Outcomes."

Am J Clin Nutr 89/5 (2009):1488s-1493j.

http://care.diabetesjournals.org/content/29/8/1866.long

Mexican Pima diet:
http://care.diabetesjournals.org/content/16/1/369.full.pdf

Fine AM, Yates D. Epigenetics and the autosomal DNA of human populations: Clinical perspectives and personal genome tests. *Int'l J Comm Diversity* 2014; 13(1):27-42

Sandovici I. et al. Maternal Diet and Aging Alter the Epigenetic Control of a Promoter-

Enhancer Interaction at the Hnf4A Gene in Rat Pancreatic Iislets. *Proc Natl Acad Sci USA* 108/13 (2011):5449-54.

Schultz L.C. The Dutch Hunger Winter and the Developmental Origins of Health and Disease. Proc Natl Acad Sci USA 107/39 (2010):16757-8.

Chapter 3

Gancevicience R et al. Skin anti-aging strategies. *Dermatoendocrinol* 2012 July 1;4(3):308-319.

Fusco D et al. Effects of antioxidant supplementation on the aging process. *Clin Interv Aging* 2007;2:377-87.

Ladermann J et al. Influence of Topical, Systemic and Combined Application of Antioxidants on the Barrier Properties of the Human Skin. *Skin Pharmacol Physiol.* 2016;29(1):41-6. doi: 10.1159/000441953. Epub 2016 Jan 23

Tian FF et al. Nrf2-mediated protection against UVA radiation in human skin keratinocytes. *Biosci Trends* 2011;5(1):23-9.

Ryu J, Kwon M-J, Nam T-J. Nrf2 and NF-κB Signaling Pathways Contribute to Porphyra-334-Mediated Inhibition of UVA-Induced Inflammation in Skin Fibroblasts. Jacobson PB, ed. *Marine Drugs*. 2015;13(8):4721-4732. doi:10.3390/md13084721.

Schafer M et al. Nrf2 establishes a glutathione-mediated gradient of UVB cytoprotection in the epidermis. *Genes & Dev* 2010 24:1045-1058.

Patricia OyetakinWhite, Heather Tribout, and Elma Baron, "Protective Mechanisms of Green Tea Polyphenols in Skin," *Oxidative Medicine and Cellular Longevity*, vol. 2012, Article ID 560682, 8 pages, 2012. doi:10.1155/2012/560682

Heinrich U, et al. Green tea polyphenols provide photoprotection, increase microcirculation, and modulate skin properties of women. *J Nutr.* 2011 Jun;141(6):1202-8.

Katiyar SK. Green tea prevents non-melanoma skin cancer by enhancing DNA repair. *Arch Biochem Biophys* 2011 Apr15;508(2):152-8.

Katiyar SK. et al. Green tea polyphenols prevent UV-induced immunosuppression by rapid repair of DNA damage and enhancement of nucleotide excision repair genes. *Cancer Prev Res (Phila)* 2010 Feb;3(2):179-89.

Katiyar SK et al. Green tea polyphenol treatment to human skin prevents formation of ultraviolet light B-induced pyrimidine dimers in DNA. *Clin Cancer Res* 2000 Oct;6(10):3864-9.

Bae JY et al. Bog blueberry anthocyanins alleviate photoaging in ultraviolet-B irradiation-induced human dermal fibroblasts. *Mol Nutr Food Res* 2009 Jun;53(6):726-38

Pageon H. Reconstructed skin modified by glycation of the dermal equivalent as a model for skin-aging and its potential use to evaluate anti-glycation molecules. *Exp Gerontol* 2008 Jun;43(6):584-8.

Chen L. et al Phytochemical properties and antioxidant capacities of various colored berries. *J Sci Food Agri* 2013 May 7 doi:10.1002/jsfa.6216 (Epub ahead of print)

Johnson MH et al. Anthocyanins and proanthocyandins from blueberry-blackberry fermented beverages inhibit markers of inflammation in macrophages and carbohydrate-utilizing enzymes in vitro. *Mol Nutr Food Res* 2013 Jul;57(7):1182-97.

Kolosova NG et al. Comparison of antioxidants in the ability to prevent cataract in prematurely aging OXYS rats. *Bull Exp Biol Med* 2004 Mar;137(3):249-51.

Huang C. et al. Inhibition of benzo(a)pyrene diol epoxide-induced transactivation of activated protein 1 and nuclear factor kappa B by black raspberry extracts. *Cancer Res* 2002 Dec 1;62(23):6857-63.

Bae JY et al. Bog blueberry anthocyanins alleviate photoaging in ultraviolet-B irradiation-induced human dermal fibroblasts. *Mol Nutr Food Res* 2009 Jun;53(6):726-38.

Jariyapamornkoon N et al. Inhibition of advanced glycation end products by red grape skin extract and its antioxidant activity. BMC Complement Altern Med 2013 Jul 12;13:171

Bae JY et al. Dietary compound ellagic acid alleviates skin wrinkle and inflammation induced by UV-B irradiation. *Experimental Dermatology* 2010 Aug;19(8):182-90.

Bishayee A et al. Pomegranate-mediated chemoprevention of experimental hepatocarcinogenesis involves Nrf-2-regulated antioxidant mechanism. *Carcinogenesis.* 2011 Jun;32(6):888-96.

George J et al. Synergistic growth inhibition of mouse skin tumors by pomegranate fruit extract and diallyl sulfide: evidence for inhibition of activated MAPKs/NF-kB and reduced cell proliferation. *Food Chem Toxicol* 2011 Jul;49(7):1511-20.

Park HM et al. Extract of Punica granatum inhibits skin photoaging induced by UVB irradiation. *Int J Dermatol* 2010 Mar;49(3):276-82.

Derosa G et al. Effects of n-3 PUFAs on postprandial variation of metalloproteinases and inflammatory and insulin resistance parameters in dyslipidemic patients: evaluation with euglycemic clamp and oral fat control. *J Clin Lipidol* 2012 Nov-Dec;6(6):553-64.

Li F et al. Human gut bacterial commensals are altered by addition of cruciferous vegetables in a controlled fruit and vegetable-free diet. *J Nutr* 2009 September;139(9):1685-1601.

Benno Y et al. Comparison of fecal microflora of elderly persons in rural and urban areas of Japan. *Appl Environ Microbiol* 1989 May;55(5):1100-1105.

Latreille J et al. Dietary monounsaturated fatty acids intake and risk of skin photoaging. *PLoS One* 2012;7(9):e44490.

Nagata C et al. Association of dietary fat, vegetables and antioxidant micronutrients with skin aging in Japanese women. *Br J Nutr.* 2010 May;03(10): 1493-8.

Piccardi N, Manissier P. Nutrition and nutritional supplementation. *Dermatoendocrinology.* 2009 Sep-Oct;1(5):271-274.

Unlu NZ et al. Carotenoid absorption from salad and salsa by humans is enhanced by the addition of avocado or avocado oil. *J Nutr* 2005 Mar;135(3):431-6.

Dreher ML, Davenport AJ. Hass avocado composition and potential health effects. *Crit Rev Food Sci Nutr* 2013;53(7):738-50.

Rosenblat G et al. Polyhydroxylated fatty alcohols derived from avocado suppress inflammatory response and provide non-sunscreen protection against UV-induced damage in skin cells. *Arch Dermatol Res* 2011 May;303(4):239-46.

Pilkington S, Watson R, Nicolau A, Rhodeo L. Omega-3 polyunsaturated fatty acids: phytoprotective macronutrients. *Experimental Dermatology.* 2011;20(7):537-543.

Segger D et al. Supplementation with Eskimo Skin Care improves skin elasticity in women: A pilot study. *J Dermatological Treatment* 2008:19(5):279-83.

Calder PC Mechanism of action of (n-3) fatty acids. *J Nutr* 2012 Mar;142(3):592s-599s.

Kusunoki C, et al. Omega-3 polyunsaturated fatty acid has an anti-oxidant effect via the NRF-2/HO-1 pathway in 3T3-Li adipocytes. *Biochem Biophys Res Commun* 2013 Jan 4:430(1):225-30.

Kim HH et al. Eicosapentaeoic acid inhibits UV-induced MMP-1 expression in human dermal fibroblasts. *J Lipid Res* 2005 Aug;46(8):1712-20.

Clarkson TW. The three modern faces of mercury. *Environ Health Perspect.* 2002;110(1):11-23.

Choudhury K et al. Use of skin-lightening creams. Danger from mercury. BMJ Mar 1;342:d1327.doi:10.1136/bmj.d1327

Peregrino CP et al. Mercury levels in locally manufactured Mexican skin-lightening creams. *Int J Environ Res Public Health* 2011 Jun;8(6):2516-23.

Chan TY. Inorganic mercury poisoning associated with skin-lightening cosmetic products. *Clin Toxicol* 2011 Dec;49(10):886-91.

Schager SK et al. Discovering the link between nutrition and skin aging. *Dermatoendocrinol* 2012 July 1:4(3):298-307.

Whitehead RD et al. Attractive skin coloration: harnessing sexual selection to improve diet and health. *Evol Psychol* 2012 Dec 20;10(5):842-54.

Fabian CJ, Dimler BF et al. Marine-derived omega-3 fatty acids. *Am Soc Clin Oncol Educ Book* 2013;2013:97-101.

Purba, MB et al. Skin wrinkling; can food make a difference? *J Am Coll Nutr* 2001 Feb;20(1):71-80.

Sebekova K et al. Plasma levels of advanced glycation end-products in healthy, long-term vegetarians and subjects on a Western mixed diet. *Eur J Nutr* 2001;40:275-281.

Karlic H et al. Vegetarian diet affects genes of oxidative metabolism and collagen synthesis. *Ann Nutr Metab* 2008;53(1):29-32.

Saraswat,M et al. Prevention of non-enzymic glycation of proteins by dietary agents: prospects for alleviating diabetic complications. *Br J Nutr* 2009 Jun;101(11):1714-21.

Takagi Y et al. Significance of fructose-induced protein oxidation and formation of advanced glycation end product. *J Diabetes Complications.* 1995 Apr-Jun;9(2):87-91.

Uribarri J et al. Advanced glycation end-products in foods and a practical guide to their reduction in the diet. *J Am Diet Assoc* 2010 Jun;110(6):911-16.

Gkogkolou P et al. Advanced glycation end products. *Dermatoendocrinol* 2012 Jul;4(3):259-270.

Macias-Cervantes M et al. Effect of an advanced glycation end product-restricted diet and exercise on metabolic parameters in adult overweight men. *Nutrition.* 2015 Mar;31(3):446-51

Vos M et al. Dietary fructose consumption among US children and adults: The Third National Health and Nutrition Examination Survey. *Medscape J Med* 2008; 10(7):160.

Chapter 4

Ozuguz P et al. Evaluation of serum vitamins A and E and zinc levels according to the severity of acne vulgaris. *Cutan Ocul Toxicol* 2014 Jun;33(2):99-102.

Makpol S et al. gamma-Tocotrienol prevents oxidative stress-induced telomere shortening in human fibroblasts derived from different aged individuals. *Oxid Med Cell Longev.* 2010 Jan-Feb;3(1):35-43.

Poljsak B, Dahmane R. Free radicals and extrinsic skin aging. *Dermatol Res Pract* 2012;2012:135206. Doi: 10.1155/2012/135206

Davis DR et al. Changes in USDA Food Composition Data for 43 Garden Crops, 1950-1999. *Journal of the American College of Nutrition* 2004;23(6):669-682.

Afaq F, et al. Polyphenols: skin photoprotection and inhibition of photocarcinogenesis. *Mini Rev Med Chem* 2011 Dec;11(14):1200-15.

Sharma SD at al. Dietary grape seed proanthocyanidins inhibit UVB-induced cychooxygenase-2 expression and other inflammatory mediators in UVB-exposed skin and skin tumors of SKH-1 hairless mice. *Pharm Res* 2010 Jun;27(6):1092-102.

Fine, AM. Oligomeric proanthocyanidin complexes: history, structure, and phytopharmaceutical applications. *Altern Med Rev* 2000 Apr;5(2):144-51.

Lee D et al. Clinical evidence of effects of Lactobacillus plantarum HY7714 on skin aging; a randomized, double blind, placebo controlled study. *J Microbiol Biotechnol* 2015;25(6).

Kim HM et al. Oral administration of Lactobacillus plantarum HY7714 protects hairless mouse against ultraviolet B-induced photoaging *J Microbiol Biotechnol* 2014 Nov 28;24(11):1583-91.

Parodi A et al. Small intestinal bacterial overgrowth in rosacea: clinical effectiveness of its eradication. *Clin Gastroenterol Hepatol.* 2008 Jul;6(7):759-64.

Bowe W et al. Acne vulgaris, probiotics and the gut-brain-skin axis - back to the future? *Gut Pathog.* 2011; 3(1):1.

American Academy of Dermatology, Schaumburg, 2014. http://www.aad.org/stories-and-news/news-releases/could-probiotics-be-the-next-big-thing-in-acne-and-rosacea-treatments.

Groeger D, O'Mahony L, Murphy EE, et al. *Bifidobacterium infantis* 35624 modulates host inflammatory processes beyond the gut. *Gut Microbes.* 2013;4(4):325-339.

Gueniche A, Philippe D, Bastien P, et al. Randomised double-blind placebo-controlled study of the effect of *Lactobacillus paracasei* NCC 2461 on skin reactivity. *Benef Microbes.* 2014;5(2):137-145.

Nesaretnam K et al. Tocotrienols: inflammation and cancer.

Ann N Y Acad Sci. 2011 Jul;1229:18-22.

Keileh M. et al. Role of NF-kappaB in the anti-inflammatory effects of tocotrienols *J Am Coll Nutr.* 2010 Jun;29(3 Suppl):334S-339S.

Makpol S et al. Comparative effects of biodynes, tocotrienol-rich fraction, and tocopherol in enhancing collagen synthesis and inhibiting collagen degradation in stress-induced premature senescence model of human diploid fibroblasts. *Oxid Med Cell Longev.* 2013;2013:298574. doi: 10.1155/2013/298574. Epub 2013 Dec 14

Soeur J et al. Skin resistance to oxidative stress induced by resveratrol: from Nrf2 activation to GSH biosynthesis. *Free Radic Biol Med.* 2015 Jan;78:213-23.

Buonocore D et al. Resveratrol-procyanidin blend: nutraceutical and antiaging efficacy evaluated in a placebocontrolled, double-blind study *Clin Cosmet Investig Dermatol.* 2012; 5: 159–165.

Ungvari Z et al. Mitochondrial Protection by Resveratrol *Exerc Sport Sci Rev.* 2011;39(3):128-132.

Gibillini L et al. Natural Compounds Modulating Mitochondrial Functions *Evid Based Complement Alternat Med.* 2015; 2015: 527209.

Singh M et al. New Enlightenment of Skin Cancer Chemoprevention through Phytochemicals:*In Vitro* and *In Vivo* Studies and the Underlying MechanismsBiomed *Res Int.* 2014; 2014: 243452.

Shi J, Yu J, Pohoorly JE, Kakuda Y. Polyphenolics in grape seeds-biochemistry and functionality. *J Med Food* 2003 6(4):291-9.

Binic I et al. Skin Ageing: Natural Weapons and Strategies. *Evidence-Based Complementary and Alternative Medicine* 2013

Daley C et al. A review of fatty acid profiles and antioxidant content in grass-fed and grain-fed beef *Nutr J.* 2010; 9: 10

Mohajeri S et al. Review of evidence for dietary influences on atopic dermatitis Skin Therapy Lett. 2014 Jul-Aug;19(4):5-7.

Storey A et al. Eicosapentaenoic acid and docosahexaenoic acid reduce UVB- and TNF-alpha-induced IL-8 secretion in keratinocytes and UVB-induced IL-8 in fibroblasts. *J Invest Dermatol.* 2005;124:248–55

Shahbakhti H et al. Influence of eicosapentaenoic acid, an omega-3 fatty acid, on ultraviolet-B generation of prostaglandin-E-2 and proinflammatory cytokines interleukin-1 beta, tumor necrosis factor-alpha, inter-leukin-6 and interleukin-8 in human skin in vivo. *Photochem Photobiol.* 2004;80:231–5

Cho S. The Role of Functional Foods in Cutaneous Anti-aging *J Lifestyle Med*. 2014 Mar; 4(1): 8–16.

Calder P. Mechanisms of Action of (n-3) Fatty Acids *J Nutr.* 2012 Mar;142(3):592S-599S.

Boelsma E et al. Nutritional skin care: health effects of micronutrients and fatty acids

Am J Clin Nutr. 2001 May;73(5):853-64

Segger D et al. Supplementation with Eskimo Skin Care improves skin elasticity in women. A pilot study .*J Dermatolog Treat.* 2008;19(5):279-83.

Asserin J et al. The effect of oral collagen peptide supplementation on skin moisture and the dermal collagen network: evidence from an *ex vivo* model and randomized, placebo-controlled clinical trials *J Cosmet Dermatol.* 2015 Sep 12. doi: 10.1111/jocd.12174. [Epub ahead of print

Gupta S et al. Discovery of Curcumin, a Component of the Golden Spice, and Its Miraculous Biological Activities *Clin Exp Pharmacol Physiol.* 2012 Mar; 39(3): 283–299.

Heng MC. Curcumin targeted signaling pathways: basis for anti-photoaging and anti-carcinogenic therapy. *Int J Dermatol.* 2010;49:608–22

Schagen S et al. Discovering the link between nutrition and skin aging *Dermatoendocrinol.* 2012 Jul 1; 4(3): 298–307.

Gupta S et al. Therapeutic Roles of Curcumin: Lessons Learned from Clinical Trials *AAPS J.* 2013 Jan; 15(1): 195–218.

Rhie G et al.. Aging- and photoaging-dependent changes of enzymic and nonenzymic antioxidants in the epidermis and dermis of human skin *in vivo. J. Investig. Dermatol.* 2001;117:1212–1217

Makpol S et al. Modulation of collagen synthesis and its gene expression in human skin fibroblasts by tocotrienol-rich fraction *Arch Med Sci.* 2011 Oct; 7(5): 889–895.

Rinnethaler M et al. Oxidative Stress in Aging Human Skin *Biomolecules.* 2015 Jun; 5(2): 545–589.

Godic A The Role of Antioxidants in Skin Cancer Prevention and Treatment *Oxid Med Cell Longev.* 2014; 2014: 860479.

Gkogkolou P et al. Advanced glycation end products: Key players in skin aging? *Dermatoendocrinol.* 2012 Jul 1; 4(3): 259–270.

Heng MC Curcumin targeted signaling pathways: basis for anti-photoaging and anti-carcinogenic therapy. Int J Dermatol. 2010 Jun;49(6):608-22

Gegotek A et al. The role of transcription factor Nrf2 in skin cells metabolism *Arch Dermatol Res.* 2015; 307(5): 385–396

Thankapazham RC et al. Beneficial role of curcumin in skin diseases. *Adv Exp Med Biol.* 2007;595:343-57.

Thankapazham RC et al. Skin regenerative potentials of curcumin *Biofactors* 2013 Jan-Feb;39(1):141-9.

RE De et al. Oxygenated-Blood Colour Change Thresholds for Perceived Facial Redness, Health, and Attractiveness *PLoS One.* 2011; 6(3): e17859.

Tundis R et al. Potential role of natural compounds against skin aging *Curr Med Chem.* 2015;22(12):1515-38.

Fridlender M et al. Plant derived substances with anti-cancer activity: from folklore to practice *Front Plant Sci.* 2015; 6: 799.

Aggerwal B et al. Curcumin: an orally bioavailable blocker of TNF and other pro-inflammatory biomarkers *Br J Pharmacol.* 2013 Aug; 169(8): 1672–1692.

Reuter S et al. Epigenetic changes induced by curcumin and other natural compounds *Genes Nutr.* 2011 May; 6(2): 93–108

Sonovane K et al. Topical curcumin-based cream is equivalent to dietary curcumin in skin cancer model. *J Skin Canc* 2012;1-9, Doi:10.1155'2012147863.

Schafer M et al. Nrf2 establishes a glutathione-mediated gradient of UVB cytoprotection in the epidermis. *Genes and Devel* 2010;24:1045-1058

Camera E et al.. Astaxanthin, canthaxanthin and beta-carotene differently affect UVA-induced oxidative damage and expression of oxidative stress-responsive enzymes. Exp Dermatol. 2009 Mar;18(3):222-31. Epub 2008 Sep

Yamashita, E. Beauty From Within: A Synergistic Combination Of Astaxanthin And Tocotrienol For Beauty Supplements (2002) Cosmetic Benefit of Dietary Supplements Containing Astaxanthin and Tocotrienol on Human Skin. Food Style 21 6(6):112-17.

Bruns D et al. Nrf2 Signaling and the Slowed Aging Phenotype: Evidence from Long-Lived Models *Oxid Med Cell Longev.* 2015; 2015: 732596.

Lewis K et al. Nrf2, a Guardian of Healthspan and Gatekeeper of Species Longevity *Integr Comp Biol.* 2010 Nov; 50(5): 829–843.

Anthonavage M et al. Effects of Oral Supplementation With Methylsulfonylmethane on Skin Health and Wrinkle Reduction *Natural Medicine Journal* 2015 Nov; 7(11)

Stvolinkstii SL et al. Protective effect of carnosine on Cu,Zn-superoxide dismutase during impaired oxidative metabolism in the brain in vivo. *Bull Exp Biol Med.* 2003 Feb;135(2):130-2.

Hipkiss AR On the enigma of carnosine's anti-ageing actions.

Exp Gerontol. 2009 Apr;44(4):237-42

Yamakoski J, Sano A, Tokutake S, Salito M et al. Oral intake of proanthocyanidin-rich extract from grape seeds improves chloasma. *Phytother Res* 2004 Nov;18(11):895-9.

Mantena SK, Katiyar SK. Grape seed proanthocyanidins inhibit UV-radiation-induced oxidative stress and activation of MAPL and JF-kappaB signaling in human epidermal keratinocytes. *Free Radic Biol Med* 2006 May:40(9):1603-14.

Vaid M, Prasad R, Singh T, Jones V, Katiyar SK. Grape seed proanthocyanidins reactivate silenced tumor suppressor genes in human skin cancer cells by targeting epigenetic regulators. *Toxicol Appl Pharmacol* 2012 Aug 14;263(1):122-30.

Proksch E et al. Oral supplementation of specific collagen peptides has beneficial effects on human skin physiology: a double-blind, placebo-controlled study. *Skin Pharmacol Physiol.* 2014;27(1):47-55.

Tominaga K, Hongo N, Karoto M, Yamashita E. Cosmetic benefits of astaxanthin on human subjects. *Acta Biochim Pol* 2012;59(1):43-7.

Sugarnuma, K., Nakajima, H., Ohtsuki, M., and Imokawa, G.. Astaxanthin attenuates the UVA-induced up-regulation of matrix-metalloprotein-1 and skin fibroblast elastase in human dermal fibroblasts. J Dermatol Sci 2010 May;58(2);136-42.

Palombo P et al. Beneficial Long-Term Effects of Combined Oral/Topical Antioxidant Treatment with the Carotenoids Lutein and Zeaxanthin on Human Skin: A Double-Blind, Placebo-Controlled Study. *Skin Pharmacol Physiol* 2007;20:199–210

Park K. Role of micronutrients in skin health and function. *Biomol Ther* 2015 May;23(3);207-217.

Cho S. The role of functional foods in cutaneous anti-aging. *J Lifestyle Med* 2014 Mar 4(1):8-16.

E. Patterson et al. Health Implications of High Dietary Omega-6 Polyunsaturated Fatty Acids. *Journal of Nutrition and Metabolism*, vol. 2012, Article ID 539426, 16 pages, 2012. doi:10.1155/2012/539426

Blasbalg T et al. Changes in consumption of omega-3 and omega-6 fatty acids in the United States during the 20th century *Am J Clin Nutr*. 2011 May; 93(5): 950–962.

Black HS et al. The potential of omega-3 fatty acids in the prevention of non-melanoma skin cancer. *Cancer Detect Prev.* 2006;30(3):224-32.

Chen AC et al. Oral and systemic phytoprotection. *Photodermatol Photoimmune Photomed* 2014 Apr-Jun;30(2-3):102-11.

Chapter 5

DeLuca C et al. Monitoring antioxidant defenses and free radical production in space-flight, aviation and railway engine operators, for the prevention and treatment of oxidative stress, immunological impairment, and pre-mature cell aging. *Toxicol Ind Health* 2009 25: 259-267.

Sokal K et al. Earthing the human body influences physiologic processes *J Altern Complement Med.* 2011 Apr;17(4):301-8.

Oschman J et al. The effects of grounding (earthing) on inflammation, the immune response, wound healing, and prevention and treatment of chronic inflammatory and autoimmune diseases *J Inflamm Res.* 2015; 8: 83–96.

Dhillon G et al. Triclosan: Current Status, Occurrence, Environmental Risks and Bioaccumulation Potential *Int J Environ Res Public Health.* 2015 May; 12(5): 5657–5684.

Vandenburg L et al. Hormones and Endocrine-Disrupting Chemicals: Low-Dose Effects and Nonmonotonic Dose Responses *Endocr Rev.* 2012 Jun; 33(3): 378–455.

Allen JG et al. Exposure to flame retardant chemicals on commercial airplanes *Environ Health.* 2013 Feb 16;12:17. doi: 10.1186/1476-069X-12-17

Chapter 6

http://www.ewg.org/research/body-burden-pollution-newborns. Accessed 12/18/15

Poljsak B et al. Free radicals and extrinsic skin aging. *Dermatol Res Pract* 2012:2012:135206. Doi:10.1155/2012.135206

Vierkotter A et al. Airborne particle exposure and extrinsic skin aging. *J Invest Dermatol* 2010;130:2719-2726.

Roberts WE. Pollution as a risk factor for the development of melisma and other skin disorders of facial hyperpigmentation- is there a case to be made? *J Drugs Dermatol* 2015 Apr;14(4):337-41.

Bowe W, Logan A. Acne vulgaris, probiotics and the gut-brain-skin axis - back to the future? *Gut Pathog.* 2011; 3(1): 1.

Bischoff S, et al. Intestinal permeability – a new target for disease prevention and therapy. *BMC Gastroenterol.* 2014; 14: 189.

Nakamura M. Environment-induced lentigines: formation of solar lentigines beyond ultraviolet radiation? *Exp Dermatol.* 2015 Mar; doi: 10.111/exd. 12690

Krutmann J et al. Pollution and skin: from epidemiological and mechanistic studies to clinical implications. *J Dermatol Sci* 2014 76:163-168.

Hodges R et al. Modulation of Metabolic Detoxification Pathways Using Foods and Food-Derived Components: A Scientific Review with Clinical Application *Journal of Nutrition and Metabolism* Volume 2015 (2015)

Salem MB et al. Pharmacological Studies of Artichoke Leaf Extract and Their Health Benefits. *Plant Foods Hum Nutr.* 2015 Dec;70(4):441-53.

Krajka-Kuzniak V et al. Betanin, a beetroot component, induces nuclear factor erythroid-2-related factor 2-mediated expression of detoxifying/antioxidant enzymes in human liver cell lines. *Br J Nutr.* 2013 Dec;110(12):2138-49.

Elegbede JA et al. Effects of anticarcinogenic monterpenes on phase II hepatic metabolizing enzymes. *Carcinogenesis.* 1993 Jun;14(6): 1221-3.

Rana SV et al. Garlic in health and disease. *Nutr Res Rev.* 2011 Jun;24(1):60-71.

Chevallier A. The Encyclopedia of Medicinal Plants 1996 Dorling Kindersley London, GB.

Talafay P. Sulforaphane mobilizes cellular defenses that protect skin against damage by UV radiation Proc Natl Acad Sci U S A. 2007 Oct 30; 104(44): 17500–17505

Noh C. et al. The Synergistic Upregulation of Phase II Detoxification Enzymes by Glucosinolate Breakdown Products in Cruciferous Vegetables *Toxicology and Applied Pharmacology* Volume 174, Issue 2, 15 July 2001, Pages 146–152.

Rondanelli M et al. Health-promoting properties of artichoke in preventing cardiovascular disease by its lipidic and glycemic-reducing action. *Monaldi Arch Chest Dis* 2013;80(1):17-26.

Crinnion W. Sauna as a valuable clinical tool for cardiovascular, autoimmune, toxicant-induced and other chronic health problems. *Altern Med Rev* 2011;16(3):215-225.

Genuis S, Birkholz D, Rodushkin I, Beesoon S. Blood, urine, and sweat (BUS) study: monitoring and elimination of bioaccumulated toxic elements. *Arch Environ Contam Toxicol* 61(2):344-357.

Kowatzki D et al. Effect of regular sauna on epidermal barrier function and stratum corneum water-holding capacity in vivo in humans: a controlled study. *Dermatology* 2009;217(2):173-80.

Lee J, Roh, M, Lee, K. Effects of infrared radiation on skin photo-aging and pigmentation. *Yonsei Med J* 2006;47(4):485-490.

Chapter 7

O'Donovan A et al. Stress appraisals and cellular aging: a key role for anticipatory threat in the relationship between psychological stress and telomere length. *Brain Behav Immun* 2012;26(4):573-579.

McGraty R.(2004). Clinical Applications of Bioelectromagnetic Medicine. Rosch PJ and Markov MS (Ed.) New York, NY: Marcel Dekker.

Sokal K et al. Earthing the human body influences physiologic processes *J Altern Complement Med.* 2011 Apr;17(4):301-8.

Oschman J et al. The effects of grounding (earthing) on inflammation, the immune response, wound healing, and prevention and treatment of chronic inflammatory and autoimmune diseases *J Inflamm Res.* 2015; 8: 83–96.

Chevalier G Earthing (grounding) the human body reduces blood viscosity-a major factor in cardiovascular disease. *J Altern Complement Med.* 2013 Feb;19(2):102-10.

Qing L. Effect of forest bathing trips on human immunofunction. *Environ Health Prev Med* 2010 Jan;15(1):9-17.

Ghaly M et al. The biologic effects of grounding the human body during sleep as measured by cortisol levels and subjective reporting of sleep, pain, and stress *J Altern Complement Med.* 2004 Oct;10(5):767-76.

Epel ES et al. Accelerated telomere shortening in response to life stress. *Proc Natl Acad Sci U S A.* 2004 Dec 7;101(49):17312-5

https://www.tm.org/benefits-of-meditation. Accessed 1/22/16

Epel E et al. Can meditation slow rate of cellular aging? Cognitive stress, mindfulness, and telomeres *Ann N Y Acad Sci.* 2011 Mar 15.

Kaliman P et al. Rapid changes in histone deacetylases and inflammatory gene expression in expert meditators. *Psychoneuroendocrinology.* 2014 Feb;40:96-107.

Rubin M et al. Your Skin, Younger. Cumberland House. 2010

Leung MK et al. Increased gray matter volume in the right angular and posterior parahippocampal gyri in loving-kindness meditators. *Soc Cogn Affect Neurosci.* 2013 Jan;8(1):34-9. doi: 10.1093/scan/nss076. Epub 2012 Jul 18

Hoge EA et al. Loving-Kindness Meditation practice associated with longer telomeres in women. *Brain Behav Immun.* 2013 Aug;32:159-63. doi: 10.1016/j.bbi.2013.04.005. Epub 2013 Apr 19

Bankard J. Training Emotion Cultivates Morality: How Loving-Kindness Meditation Hones Compassion and Increases Prosocial Behavior. *J Relig Health.* 2015 Dec;54(6):2324-43. doi: 10.1007/s10943-014-9999-8.

Streeter C et al. Effects of Yoga Versus Walking on Mood, Anxiety, and Brain GABA Levels: A Randomized Controlled MRS *Study J Altern Complement Med.* 2010 Nov; 16(11): 1145–1152.

Slominski A. A nervous breakdown in the skin: stress and the epidermal barrier. *J Clin Invest* 2007;117:3166-169.

Oyetakin-White P et al. Does poor sleep quality affect skin aging? *Clin Exp Dermatol* 2015 Jan:40(1):17-22.

Slominski A et al. Local Melatoninergic System as the Protector of Skin Integrity *Int J Mol Sci.* 2014 Oct; 15(10): 17705–17732.

Park B et al. The physiological effects of *Shinrin-yoku* (taking in the forest atmosphere or forest bathing): evidence from field experiments in 24 forests across Japan. *Environ Health Prev Med.* 2010 Jan; 15(1): 18–26.

Miyazaki Y et al. Forest Medicine Research in Japan. *Japanese Journal of Hygeine* 2014;69(2):122-135.

Goon JA et al. Effect of Tai Chi exercise on DNA damage, antioxidant enzymes, and oxidative stress in middle-age adults. *J Phys Act Health.* 2009 Jan;6(1):43-54

Irwin M et al. Tai Chi, Cellular Inflammation, and Transcriptome Dynamics in Breast Cancer Survivors With Insomnia: A Randomized Controlled *Trial J Natl Cancer Inst Monogr.* 2014 Nov; 2014(50): 295–301

Ren H et al. Epigenetic Changes in Response to Tai Chi Practice: A Pilot Investigation of DNA Methylation Marks *Evid Based Complement Alternat Med.* 2012

Niles H et al. Functional Genomics in the Study of Mind-Body Therapies *Ochsner J.* 2014 Winter; 14(4): 681–695.

Huang TL et al. A comprehensive review of the psychological effects of brainwave entrainment. *Altern Ther Health Med* 2009 Sep-Oct;14(5):38-50.

Chaieb L et al. Auditory Beat Stimulation and its Effects on Cognition and Mood States *Front Psychiatry.* 2015; 6: 70.

Kaliman P et al. Rapid changes in histone deacetylases and inflammatory gene expression in expert meditators. *Psychoneuroendocrinology.* 2014 Feb;40:96-107.

Turakitwanakan W et al. Effects of mindfulness meditation on serum cortisol of medical students. *J Med Assoc Thai.* 2013 Jan;96 Suppl 1:S90-5.

Vollestad J et al. Mindfulness- and acceptance-based interventions for anxiety disorders: a systematic review and meta-analysis. *Br J Clin Psychol.* 2012 Sep;51(3):239-60.

Brand S et al. Influence of mindfulness practice on cortisol and sleep in long-term and short-term meditators *Neuropsychobiology.* 2012;65(3):109-18.

Kimata H. Elevation of testosterone and reduction of transepidermal water loss by viewing a humorous film by elderly patients with atopic dermatitis. *Acta Medica (Hradec Kralove).* 2007;50(2):135-7.

Eppley KR et al. Differential effects of relaxation techniques on trait anxiety: a meta-analysis *J Clin Psychol.* 1989 Nov;45(6):957-74.

Andrade C et al. Prayer and healing: A medical and scientific perspective on randomized controlled trials *Indian J Psychiatry.* 2009 Oct-Dec; 51(4): 247–253.

http://news.harvard.edu/gazette/story/2011/01/eight-weeks-to-a-better-brain/ accessed 12/13/15

Chapter 8

Ford ES et al. Trends in outpatient visits for insomnia, sleep apnea, and prescriptions for sleep medications among US adults: findings from the National Ambulatory Medical Care Survey 1999-2010. Sleep. 2014;37(8):1283-1293. doi:10.5665/sleep.3914.

Carroll JE, et al. Partial sleep deprivation activates the DNA damage response (DDR) and the senescence-associated secretory phenotype (SASP) in aged adult humans. *Brain Behav Immun* 2016 Jan;51:223-9.

Axelsson J et al. Beauty sleep: experimental study on the perceived health and attractiveness of sleep deprived people *BMJ.* 2010; 341: c6614.

Povoa G et al. Growth Hormone System: skin interactions *An Bras Dermatol.* 2011;86(6):1159-6.

Chervin R et al. The Face of Sleepiness: Improvement in Appearance after Treatment of Sleep Apnea *J Clin Sleep Med.* 2013 Sep; 9(9): 845–852.

Hirschkowitz H et al. National Sleep Foundation's updated sleep duration recommendations: final report. *Sleep Health* 2015 Dec;1(4):233-243.

http://www.ninds.nih.gov/disorders/brain_basics/understanding_sleep.htm accessed 11/21/15

Yarrow K. The Sleep Industry: Why We're paying big bucks for something that's free. *Time* Jan 2013.

Vriend J et al. The Keap1-Nrf2-antioxidant response element pathway: a review of its regulation by melatonin and the proteasome. *Mol Cell Endocrinol.* 2015 Feb 5;401:213-20.

Tan D et al. Melatonin as a Potent and Inducible Endogenous Antioxidant: Synthesis and Metabolism. *Molecules* 2015;20(10):18886-18906.

Cho W et al. Effects of artificial light at night on human health: A literature review of observational and experimental studies applied to exposure assessment. *Chronobiol Int.* 2015 Sep 16:1-17

Karadaq E. Effects of aromatherapy on sleep quality and anxiety of patients *Nurs Crit Care.* 2015 Jul 27. doi: 10.1111/nicc.12198. [Epub ahead of print

Lillhei HS et al. A systemic review of the effect of inhaled essential oils on sleep. *J Altern Complement Med* 2014 Jun;20(6):441-51.

Slominski A et al. Local Melatoninergic System as the Protector of Skin Integrity *Int J Mol Sci.* 2014 Oct; 15(10): 17705–17732.

Becker PM. Hypnosis in the management of sleep disorders. *Sleep Med Clin.* 2015 Mar;10(1):85-92

Statland BE et al. Serum caffeine half-lives. Healthy subjects vs. patients having alcoholic hepatic disease. *Am J Clin Pathol.* 1980 Mar;73(3):390-3.

http://www.starbucks.com/menu/drinks/brewed-coffee/pike-place-roast accessed 11/24/15

Hillert L et al. The Effects of 884 MHz GSM Wireless Communication Signals on Self-reported Symptom and Sleep (EEG)- An Experimental Provocation Study. (2007). *Bioelectromagnetics.* 3(7), 1148-1150.

K. Mann et al Effects of Pulsed High-Frequency Electromagnetic Fields on Human Sleep_2006 *Neuropsychobiology.* 33, 41-47.

Shiller H et al. Sedating effects of Humulus lupulus L. extracts.

Phytomedicine. 2006 Sep;13(8):535-41

http://cms.herbalgram.org/commissione/Monographs/Monograph0201.html. Accessed11/24/15

Weeks BS. Formulations of dietary supplements and herbal extracts for relaxation and anxiolytic action: Relarian. *Med Sci Monit.* 2009 Nov;15(11):RA256-62.

Sarris J et al. Plant-based medicines for anxiety disorders, part 2: a review of clinical studies with supporting preclinical evidence.

CNS Drugs. 2013 Apr;27(4):301-19

Laklan H et al. Nutritional and herbal supplements for anxiety and anxiety-related disorders: systematic review Nutr J. 2010; 9: 42.

Sarris J et al. Kava and St John's Wort: current evidence for use in mood and anxiety disorders. *J Altern Complement Med* 2009 Aug;15(8):827-36.

Melancon MO et al. Exercise and sleep in aging: emphasis on serotonin *Pathol Biol (Paris).* 2014 Oct;62(5):276-83.

L-Tryptophan. Monograph. *Altern Med Rev.* 2006 Mar;11(1):52-6.

Bent S et al. Valerian for Sleep: A Systematic Review and Meta-Analysis *Am J Med.* 2006 Dec; 119(12): 1005–1012.

Han D et al. Wound Healing Activity of Gamma-Aminobutyric Acid (GABA) in Rats. *J. Microbiol. Biotechnol.* 2007 ; 17(10): 1661-1669

http://www.gallup.com/poll/166553/less-recommended-amount-sleep.aspx accessed 11/10/15.

Plante D et al. Reduced γ-Aminobutyric Acid in Occipital and Anterior Cingulate Cortices in Primary Insomnia: a Link to Major Depressive Disorder? Neuropsychopharmacology. 2012 May; 37(6): 1548–1557

Oyetakin-White P et al. Does poor sleep quality affect skin ageing? *Clin Exp Dermatol.* 2015 Jan;40(1):17-22.

Altemus M et al. Stress-induced changes in skin barrier function in healthy women *J Invest Dermatol.* 2001 Aug;117(2):309-17

Black D et al. Mindfulness Meditation and Improvement in Sleep Quality and Daytime Impairment Among Older Adults With Sleep Disturbances A Randomized Clinical Trial *JAMA Intern Med.* 2015;175(4):494-501

http://www.ehhi.org/reports/cellphones/cell_phone_report_EHHI_Feb201
2.pdf accessed 11/28/15

Gooley J et al. Exposure to Room Light before Bedtime Suppresses
Melatonin Onset and Shortens Melatonin Duration in Humans *J Clin
Endocrinol Metab.* 2011 Mar; 96(3): E463–E472

Chang AM et al. Evening use of light-emitting eReaders negatively affects
sleep, circadian timing, and next-morning alertness *Proc Natl Acad Sci U S A.*
2015 Jan 27; 112(4): 1232–1237.

Holzman D. What's in a Color? The Unique Human Health Effects of Blue
Light *Environ Health Perspect* 2010; 118:A22-A27.

Halonen J et al. Associations between Nighttime Traffic Noise and Sleep:
The Finnish Public Sector Study *Environ Health Perspect 2012;120(10):*

Chapter 9

http://www.cdc.gov/biomonitoring/Parabens_BiomonitoringSummary.html
accessed 4/24/16

http://www.fda.gov/Cosmetics/ProductsIngredients/Products/ucm137224.h
tm#expanalyses accessed 3/30/2015

Al-Saleh I[1], Al-Enazi S, Shinwari N.Assessment of lead in cosmetic
products. *Regul Toxicol Pharacol* 2009 Jul;54(2):105-13.

Chan TY. Inorganic mercury poisoning associated with skin-lightening
cosmetic products. *Clin Toxicol (Phila).* 2011 Dec;49(10):886-91.

Sainio EL et al. Metals and arsenic in eye shadows *Contact Dermatitis.* 2000
Jan;42(1):5-10.

Janui NR et al. Systemic uptake of diethyl phthalate, dibutyl phthalate, and
butyl paraben following whole-body topical application and reproductive
and thyroid hormone levels in humans. *Environ Sci Technol.* 2007 Aug
1;41(15):5564-70.

http://www.cancer.org/cancer/cancerbasics/lifetime-probability-of-
developing-or-dying-from-cancer accessed 3/18/16

Woodruff TJ, et al. Environmental chemicals in pregnant women in the United States: NHANES 2003-2004. *Environ Health Perspectives* 2011(119):878-885.

Konduracka E et al. Relationship between everyday use cosmetics and female breast cancer. *Pol Arch Med Wewn.* 2014;124(5):264-9.

Khanna S, et al. Exposure to parabens at the concentration of maximal proliferative response increases migratory and invasive activity of human breast cancer cells in vitro. *J Appl Toxicol* 2014 Sep;34(9):1051-9.

http://cehr.neihs.nih.gov/chemicals/bisphenol/BPADraftbriefVF_04_04_08/pdf.

The Endocrine Society. Endocrine-Disrupting Chemicals. http://www.endo-society.org/journals/ScientificStatements/upload/EDC_Scientific_Statement.pdf. Accessed July 6, 2010.

Legler J, Fletcher T, Govarts E. et al. Obesity, diabetes, and associated costs of exposure to endocrine-disrupting chemicals in the European Union. *J Clin Endocriol Metab* 2015;100(4):1278-88.

Attina TM, et al. Exposure to endocrine-disrupting chemicals in the USA: a population-based disease burden and cost analysis *Lancet Diabetes Endocrinol.* 2016 Oct 17. pii: S2213-8587(16)30275-3. doi: 10.1016/S2213-8587(16)30275-3.

Vogel S. The politics of plastics: The making and unmaking of bisphenol A "safety". *Am J Public Health.* 2009;99(suppl 3):s559-s566.

Yang YJ, Hong YC, Oh SY, et al. Bisphenol A exposure is associated with oxidative stress and inflammation in postmenopausal women. *Environ Res.* 2009;109(6):797-801.

http://www.breastcancerfund.org/assets/pdfs/tips-fact-sheets/bpa-abstracts.pdf accessed 9/11/16

Hagobian T. et al. Randomized Intervention Trial to Decrease Bisphenol A Urine Concentrations in Women: Pilot Study *J Womens Health (Larchmt).* 2016 Oct 11. [Epub ahead of print

Paulose T et al. Estrogens in the wrong place at the wrong time: Fetal BPA exposure and mammary cancer *Reprod Toxicol.* 2015 Jul;54:58-65.

Seachrist DD et al. A review of the carcinogenic potential of bisphenol A. *Reprod Toxicol.* 2016 Jan;59:167-82

Todd H et al. Randomized Intervention Trial to Decrease Bisphenol A Urine Concentrations in Women: Pilot Study *Journal of Women's Health.* October 2016, ahead of print. doi:10.1089/jwh.2016.5746.

NTP (National Toxicology Program) (1989). NTP Technical Report on the Toxicology and Carcinogenesis Studies of Hydroquinone (CAS No. 123-31-9) in F344/N Rats and B6C3F1 Mice (Gavage Studies). National Toxicology Program. NTP TR 366 # 90-2821, Department of Health and Human Services, Washington, DC.

McGregor D. Hydroquinone: an evaluation of the human risks from its carcinogenic and mutagenic properties. *Crit Rev Toxicol.* 2007;37(10):887-914.

Kumar M, Chauhan LK, Paul BN, et al. GSTM1, GSTT1 and GSTP1 polymorphism in north Indian population and its influence on the hydroquinone-induced in vitro genotoxicity. *Toxicol Mech Methods.* 2009;19(1):59-65.

Westerhof W, Kooyers TJ. Hydroquinone and its analogues in dermatology- a potential health risk. *J Cosmet Dermatol.* 2005;4(2):55-59.

Bandyopadhyay D. Topical treatment of melasma. *Indian J Dermatol.* 2009;54(4):303-309.

Houlihan J, Brody C, Schwan B. Environmental Working Group. Not Too Pretty—Phthalates, Beauty Products & the FDA. www.safecosmetics.org/downloads/NotTooPretty_report.pdf. Accessed July 6, 2010.

Main MK. Human breast milk contamination with phthalates and alterations of endogenous reproductive hormones in infants three months of age. *Environmental Health Perspectives.* 2006;114(2):270-276.

Swan SH. Environmental phthalate exposure in relation to reproductive outcomes and other health endpoints in humans. *Environ Res.* 2008;108(2):177-184.

Meeker JD, Calafet AM, Houser R. Phthalates associated with reduced steroid hormone levels in men. *J Androl.* 2009;30(3):2887-2897.

Colon I. Identification of phthalates esters in the serum of young Puerto Rican girls with premature breast development. *Environ Health Perspect.* 2004;112(10):A 541-543.

Janjua NR. Systemic uptake of diethyl phthalate, dibutyl phthalate, and butyl paraben following whole-body topical application and reproductive and thyroid hormone levels in humans. *Environ. Sci. Technol.* 41, 15 (2007): 5564-5570.

Miller D. Estrogenic activity of phenolic additives determined by an in vitro yeast bioassay. *Environmental Health Perspectives.* 2001;109:133-138.

Darbre PD. Concentrations of parabens in human breast tumours. *Journal of Applied Toxicology.* 2004;24:5-13.

Darbre PD, Harvey PW. Paraben esters: review of recent studies of endocrine toxicity, absorption, esterase and human exposure, and discussion of potential human health risks. *J Appl Toxicol.* 2008;28(5)561-578.

Calafat AM, Ye X, Wong LY, Bishop AM, Needham LL. 2010. Urinary concentrations of four parabens in the U.S. population: NHANES 2005–2006. *Environ. Health Perspect.* 118: 679–685.

Darbre PD et al. Parabens can enable hallmarks and characteristics of cancer in human breast epithelial cells: a review of the literature with reference to new exposure data and regulatory status. *Appl Toxicol.* 2014 Sep;34(9):925-38.

U.S. National Toxicological Program. "NTP Toxicology and Carcinogenesis Studies of Lauric Acid Diethanolamine Condensate (CAS NO. 120-40-1) in F344/N Rats and B6C3F1 Mice (Dermal Studies)." *Natl Toxicol Program Tech Rep Ser.* 480 (Jul 1999):1-200.

S. National Toxicological Program. "Toxicology and carcinogenesis studies of coconut oil acid diethanolamine condensate (CAS No. 68603-42-9) in F344/N rats and B6C3F1 mice (dermal studies)." *Natl Toxicol Program Tech Rep Ser.* 479 (Jan 2001):5-226.

European Commission. Regulation (EC) 1272/2008 , Annex VI, Table 3.2. Sep 2009. http://ecb.jrc.ec.europa.eu/classification-labelling/

De Groot A, et al. Formaldehyde-releasers in cosmetics: relationship to formaldehyde contact allergy. Part 2. Patch test relationship to formaldehyde contact allergy, experimental provocation test, amount of formaldehyde released, and assessment of risk to consumers allergic to formaldehyde. *Contact Dermatitis.* 2010;62:18-31.

De Groot A, et al. Formaldehyde-releasers in cosmetics: relationship to formaldehyde contact allergy. Part 1. Characterization, frequency and relevance of sensitization, and frequency in cosmetics. *Contact Dermatitis.* 2010;62:2-17.

Kano H, et al. Thirteen-week oral toxicity of 1,4-dioxane in rats and mice. *J Toxicol Sci.* 2008;33(2):141-153.

FDA. Cosmetic Product Manufacturers (2/95). http://www.fda.gov/ICEI/Inspections/InspectionGuides/ucm074952.htm. Accesed July 6, 2010.

Krasner SW, et al. Occurrence of disinfection byproducts in United States wastewater treatment plant effluents. *Environ Sci Technol.* 2009;43(21):8320-8325.

Kemper JM, et al. Quaternary amines as nitrosamine precursors: A role for consumer products? *Environ Sci Technol.* 2010;44(4):1224-1231.

Environmental Working Group. Not so sexy hidden chemicals in perfume and cologne. http://www.ewg.org/notsosexy. Accessed July 6, 2010.

Calafat AM, et al. Urinary Concentrations of Triclosan in the US population 2003-2004. *Environmental Health Perspectives.* 2008;116(3):303-307.

Ahn KC, et al. In vitro biologic activities of the antimicrobials triclocarban, its analogs, and triclosan in bioassay screens: bioassay receptor screens. *Environmental Health Perspectives.* 2008;116(9):1203-1210.

http://www.fda.gov/NewsEvents/Newsroom/PressAnnouncements/ucm517478.htm accessed 11/15/16

Halden R. On the need and speed of regulating triclosan and trichocarban in the United States. *Environ Sci Technol* 2014;48(7):3603-3611

Campaign for Safe Cosmetics. A poison kiss: The problem of lead in lipstick. http://www.safecosmetics.org/article.php?id=327. Accessed July 6, 2010.

FDA. Lipstick and Lead: Questions and Answers. http://www.fda.gov/Cosmetics/ProductandIngredientSafety/ProductInform ation/ucm137224.htm#q4. Accessed July 6, 2010.

http://www.fda.gov/Cosmetics/ProductsIngredients/Products/ucm137224.h tm#expnalyses accessed 3/3/15

http://www.fda.gov/Cosmetics/ProductsIngredients/Products/ucm137224.h tm#expanalyses *accessed 3/30/2015*

Regul Toxicol Pharmacol. 2009 Jul;54(2):105-13. doi: 10.1016/j.yrtph.2009.02.005. Epub 2009 Feb 27.

Woodruff TJ, et al. Environmental chemicals in pregnant women in the United States: NHANES 2003-2004. *Environ Health Perspectives* 2011(119):878-885.

Konduracka E et al. Relationship between everyday use cosmetics and female breast cancer. *Pol Arch Med Wewn.* 2014;124(5):264-9.

Whanna S, et al. Exposure to parabens at the concentration of maximal proliferative response increases migratory and invasive activity of human breast cancer cells in vitro. *J Appl Toxicol* 2014 Sep;34(9):1051-9.

Harley K et al. Reducing Phthalate, Paraben, and Phenol Exposure from Personal Care Products in Adolescent Girls: Findings from the HERMOSA Intervention Study *Environ Health Perspect*; DOI:10.1289/ehp.1510514

https://www.atsdr.cdc.gov/substances/toxsubstance.asp?toxid=25 Accessed 11/15/16

http://www.epa.gov/ttnatw01/hlthef/formalde.html accessed 4/13/2015

https://www.osha.gov/SLTC/hairsalons/index.html#health_risks accessed 4/20/15

Add -
Pomegranate oil & juice
Avocado
Bone broth
Vitamin C

MSM   p. 113-114
Grape seed extract p.117 100 mg
Resveratrol 200 mg per day (400 per da
Curcumin/tumeric 500 mg per day

Made in the USA
San Bernardino, CA
15 May 2019

35859099R00184